Change
   Your Looks,
Change
   Your Life

Change Your Looks, Change Your Life

Quick Fixes and Cosmetic Surgery Solutions for Looking Younger, Feeling Healthier, and Living Better

MICHELLE COPELAND, D.M.D., M.D.,

with ALEXANDRA S. POSTMAN

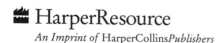 HarperResource

An Imprint of HarperCollins*Publishers*

HarperCollins books may be purchased for educational, business, or sales promotional use. For information, please write: Special Markets Department, HarperCollins Publishers Inc., 10 East 53rd Street, New York, NY 10022.

FIRST EDITION

Designed by Lindgren / Fuller Design

Printed on acid-free paper

Library of Congress Cataloging-in-Publication Data

Copeland, Dr. Michelle.
    Change your looks, change your life : quick fixes and cosmetic surgery solutions for looking younger, feeling healthier, and living better / Dr. Michelle Copeland with Alexandra S. Postman.— 1st ed.
        p.   cm.
    Includes index.
    ISBN 0-06-621373-8 (alk. paper)
    1. Surgery, Plastic—Popular works.   I. Copeland, Michelle   II. Title.

RD119 .C625   2002
617.9'5—dc21
                                                              2002024093

03 04 05 06 07 WB/RRD 10 9 8 7 6 5 4 3 2 1

To my parents, who instilled a love of learning and caring for others; to my husband, Dr. Jonathan L. Halperin, and my children, Robert and Libby, for their patience and support; and to my patients, who make it all worthwhile.

CONTENTS

PART THREE

SURGICAL SOLUTIONS

ACKNOWLEDGMENTS

This book became a reality with the assistance of many good friends, whose encouragement and guidance helped me navigate the literary maze. Delia Marshall and Candy Lee urged me on from the beginning and were there whenever I seemed to waver. My thanks as well to my literary agent, Mark Reiter, who believed in the concept from the start; to Diane Reverand, who brought it to HarperCollins; and to Susan Friedland for making it happen. Most of all, I'm deeply grateful to Alex Postman, who performed the magic of transforming clinical experience and the movements of a surgeon's hands into prose.

The Time for Change Is Now

WHAT IF?

We're a culture that imagines and embraces possibility. What if we could actually change? What if we could genuinely improve ourselves? What if we could look better than we ever have—or ever thought we could—and still remain true to ourselves? "What if?" is the idea behind this book.

Helping people imagine how their looks—and, by extension, their lives—can improve is the most challenging and rewarding part of my daily work. In my twenty years practicing as a plastic surgeon, I've met hundreds of women and men who come to my office wanting to change *something*: the violinist, spirited and vivacious as a forty-five-year-old, whose skin betrays her sixty-five years; the fifty-year-old computer executive with bags under his eyes who fears losing a deserved promotion to a younger co-worker; the thirty-seven-year-old single mom who repeatedly breaks off promising relationships because she's scared to get naked with a new partner. The effect their appearance has on their self-confidence is more than skin-deep; it has enormous impact on their emotional health, the quality of their lives, and their future outlook.

TODAY'S REVOLUTION
IN COSMETIC SURGERY

I have been privileged to witness the self-image of so many patients undergo extraordinary and dramatic changes, even after minor work. And I've come to see how cosmetic surgery can be a powerful, and empowering, tool; its reach extends beyond flattening a stomach or removing a deep-creased scowl or smoothing pitted skin. It can help to restore energy and optimism, to give that literal lift needed to make more far-reaching physical and, ultimately, psychological improvements.

Back in the early 1970s, when I was one of the few women in my class at Harvard Medical School (and the first to graduate with a dual degree in dentistry and plastic surgery), the discipline of plastic surgery was in its infancy. It had only recently shifted from its long-standing focus on reconstructive surgery (fixing cleft palates and badly broken noses, for instance) to cosmetic (or aesthetic) surgery, the practice of doing for people what nature didn't or couldn't. We who specialized in cosmetic surgery performed massive, Hollywood-style face-lifts and experimented with such new body-sculpting procedures as liposuction; the results, while encouraging, were less than stellar. As technology improved, we were able to make even more dramatic changes on patients who needed or wanted them.

Today, we have entered a kind of Golden Age of plastic and cosmetic surgery: In just the last half-decade, medical advances have greatly reduced the invasiveness, risk, pain, and recovery time of most procedures, radically transforming what the profession can do. No longer must every fix and its aftermath be anxiety-ridden, painful, or time-consuming. New techniques like these have contributed to advances in the field:

◆ Twilight sleep puts patients in a deeply relaxed state without the debilitating grogginess of general anesthesia. Patients walk out of my office on their own just a couple of hours after a procedure.

◆ Endoscopic surgery, which uses a long, thin tube attached to a video camera, allows me to perform such procedures as a forehead lift with only three tiny incisions behind the hairline, rather than the old ear-to-ear "headband" incision that leaves a nasty scar. Recovery time? Three days, versus three weeks.

◆ Liposuction, first introduced in the 1980s, has improved to the point where we can now remove large amounts of fat from all over the body, all at once, without causing the blood loss and massive bruising and swelling that used to be routine. And large-scale surgical procedures such as tummy tucks, neck lifts, and arm lifts are now often eschewed in favor of lipo, which in many cases tightens and flattens skin just as effectively with virtually no scarring.

◆ Small-incision surgery means shorter, better-placed, and quicker-to-heal scars for almost all procedures. A face-lift used to require a long, winding incision from the temple area, under the ear, and into the hairline. Now I usually opt to do a "mini-lift," requiring a much shorter, and less visible, incision. Another example: Breast reductions used to incur a three-part scar, with the longest section in the breast crease. Today, I resort to this traditional method only when breasts are far too big to support one of the smaller-scar alternatives: an incision around the nipple, or one around the nipple and down to the breast crease. Not only do smaller incisions minimize scarring, but with a quicker recovery they are good news for those who must return to normal life as quickly as possible after surgery.

◆ Many new techniques achieve superb results *without* surgery. For example, I may opt to forgo a face-lift and instead perform a series of minor procedures without putting someone under the knife. Collagen or fat injections in the face strategically plump it up; while microdermabrasion, a painless process in which a steady stream of fine crystals is sprayed at the skin, dramatically buffs and tightens the skin's surface, especially in combination with light lasers, which stimulate new collagen growth.   .

In short, what were once major surgeries are now outpatient procedures that can be done in my office, during lunchtime.

THE "ART" OF SCIENCE:
A WOMAN'S TOUCH

Scientific progress is only part of what defines my job. Over the years—and very much with the help of my patients—I've come to see that plastic surgery is an art. If I'm a scientist first, then I must be an artist second. And I learned this because I listen: My patients share their wishes and concerns; along with my fellow surgeons, I use the increasingly adaptive technology at my fingertips to express what is unique and beautiful about each person, and I attempt to do this creatively and sensitively.

Let me repeat something I just said: *I express what is unique and beautiful about each person.* That is it, in a nutshell. In recent years, surgeons have become more educated in the subtleties of beauty—real-life, individual beauty, not the cookie-cutter perfection we associate with the oft-lifted, tucked, and bobbed. And we've grown much better at "sculpting" human beings.

Why? Frankly, I think it's because of the rising number of women plastic surgeons in the field.

That sounds sexist, I know. But I can testify to how things *used* to be, and they weren't pretty. I had a hard time becoming a plastic surgeon. In the 1970s, when it came to giving women an equal chance, even Harvard was less than enlightened. On the first day of anatomy class, the professor projected on the screen a slide of a Rubenesque naked woman. Pretty much everyone but me (one of only a couple of women in the class) hooted at her voluptuous curves. Today, those former medical students are out in the world, shaping noses, recontouring thighs, enlarging or reducing breasts—in short, helping to define beauty. And many of those male surgeons tend to style *their* idea of the perfect woman—like so many Pygmalions. The problem with that? The ideal that guides men is often a far cry from female standards of beauty.

It's cliché to say that women are more empathetic and better listeners than men, but I find that female surgeons naturally take a more collaborative approach with their patients, rather than offering fatherly wisdom or intimations of male flattery. As a woman, for instance, I never create the breasts *I* want to see on a patient; I create the breasts *she* wants to see. Or scars: For a woman, a scar is ugly—a blemish that invites curiosity, rather than a badge of honor, as many men see it. So I always explore with a patient ways of mini-mizing (or altogether avoiding) scarring, a concern that I believe many of my male colleagues have overlooked for far too long.

Fortunately, many male doctors have now "got it." Increasingly more attentive and responsive, they're better able to listen to and work with a patient as a partner. In turn, patients are more likely to go into a first consul-tation with a prospective surgeon feeling empowered, and can expect cus-tomized procedures that take into account cultural, ethnic, and personal preferences.

To be a good plastic surgeon, then, it is not enough to possess know-how, manual dexterity, and framed diplomas that trumpet our qualifications. We must also be imaginative, resourceful, and respectful. To do my job well, I must make sure that the women and men who leave my office not only look better but *feel* better. And while not all doctors practice this way, I'll show in the following chapters how to hold *your* doctor to the same high standards.

All patients must have the courage to ask, "What if?" That way, they can embrace all the wonderful possibilities that plastic surgery offers.

COSMETIC WELLNESS: WHY LOOKING GOOD IS GOOD *FOR* YOU

Before I address the questions my patients invariably ask when considering surgery and the specifics of the surgery itself, please consider one more thing: Cosmetic surgery not only can help fix something that has long bothered you, but it can be the catalyst for all kinds of other improvements. Sure, your face and/or body will improve, but more to the point, your *life* will improve.

Countless times I've seen how cosmetic surgery patients, after their proce-dures, change their approach to physical well-being, and this sets off a positive domino effect that improves their mind-set, too. When a patient sees a differ-ence to her jawline or waistline, she becomes more motivated to take care of herself. Again and again I see patients embrace, post-surgery, a skin-care regi-men or workout program with new enthusiasm and dedication because the results they've sought for so long are finally visible, with more results within reasonable reach. Indeed, a physical improvement often jump-starts an entirely new approach to living.

After surgery, patients are likely to create a different look for themselves—new wardrobe, hairstyle, makeup—which, in turn, emboldens them to take important life steps such as switching careers, or beginning a new relationship, or simply feeling confident about how they look when they walk into a room. I call this happy phenomenon *cosmetic wellness.*

I'll tell you something else, which will probably surprise you: Cosmetic intervention itself can be *physically healthy.* That's right! For instance, topical treatments like microdermabrasion and laser resurfacing stimulate the skin's own cells to regenerate, tightening and invigorating skin to do what nature can no longer get it to do on its own. And liposuction has been shown to make patients not just "thinner" but actually *healthier:* A study presented at a recent conference of the American Society for Plastic Surgeons showed that women who'd undergone large-volume liposuction lowered their blood pressure and insulin level (a risk factor for diabetes). And anyone with double-D-sized breasts who has had them reduced enjoys immense relief once her back and shoulders are not being damaged by constant tugging on her frame.

Getting my patients to subscribe to cosmetic wellness is, in the end, why I do what I do. But their commitment to looking and feeling better transcends the mere physical; the more profound improvement is almost invariably psychological. How we feel about ourselves has as much impact on our overall well-being as does eating right, exercising regularly, and lowering the toxic stress levels of our jobs, relationships, and bad habits. Even nutrition gurus and health-club freaks admit that no amount of "healthy" behavior makes up for poor attitude and low self-esteem.

Best of all, cosmetic wellness—a holistic approach to physical and emotional health—is in *your* power. In fact, I'd argue (and most mental health professionals will agree) that it's your critical personal responsibility to take a farther-reaching approach to your well-being. Because when you feel good about yourself—when you're performing at your peak, and feeling fully "optimized"—then you're a better partner, lover, parent, professional, and friend.

This is why I believe plastic surgery and other cosmetic interventions are as critical a part of being healthy as are working out regularly, eating a low-fat balanced diet, taking vitamins, meditating, and getting enough sleep. Following these steps will help you to be the best you can be—top to bottom, inside and out, in every way.

That's what this book is about. Now let's talk about you.

PART ONE

Take Control of Your Looks

1 | Getting to "Yes": Making the Decision

Now that you have a sense of what cosmetic surgery can offer, let's explore why you picked up this book.

Take a long, honest look in the mirror. You can do it for real (turn on that harsh overhead light and peel off some clothing), but my bet is you've done it often enough to know what it is about your body or face that you'd like to change.

What is it, for you? Maybe you've caught sight of that wattle that blurs your chin line (or, worse, that hangs over your crisp white collar) too many times. Maybe it's the crow's-feet that grab makeup and make a spray of fright lines at the corners of your eyes. Maybe it's your nose or earlobes, both of which sag as we age. Maybe it's your "Hi Janes" (the fleshy underside of the arm that continues to wiggle after you've stopped waving hello to your friend Jane); do they make you avoid wearing your favorite sleeveless blouse or halter top? Maybe it's your breasts—how far down has gravity pulled them? Maybe it's your stomach—are you willing to expose your midriff? (Perhaps you're currently carrying too much weight, once carried too much weight and your skin just hasn't got the message yet, or were never able to pull things up and together after your last pregnancy.) Maybe it's your hips: Is there no

A-line skirt out there that can hide hips that bear witness to every Krispy Kreme you've wolfed down? Maybe it's those pesky spider veins, crisscrossing the backs of your legs like road maps of the East Coast. I could go on and on.

Perhaps you recognized yourself in one of these complaints, or more than one. If misery loves company, then at least you'll be happy to know that virtually everyone sees a problem or three when looking in the mirror.

That's the bad news. But we're positive thinkers here, and we're going to leave harsh reality behind. Instead, let's conjure that wonderful phrase again: "What if?"

CHANGE IS WITHIN YOUR POWER

What if you could wave a wand and change *just one part* of your body—what would it be? (Forget whether it's practical, reasonable, or defensible, or whether anyone—including your own judgmental self—would "approve.") Now ask yourself something else: How many times in the last week have you thought about your nose, or crow's-feet, or wattle, or saddlebags? How many times in the last day? How many times have you thought about that "flaw" in the last five years?

Now ask yourself how your life might have been different, in big ways or small, in the last five years if you hadn't been self-conscious about this part of yourself. How might your attitude about yourself have been different? How might this have had a ripple effect on the rest of your life?

The way we see ourselves and believe we're perceived by others is tied up with the way we look. Call it shallow, label it politically incorrect, swear that real beauty is on the inside . . . but, like it or not, looks matter. Beauty has always been a powerful stimulus and motivator: Throughout history, across all cultures, people have loaded themselves down with uncomfortable jewelry, submitted to body piercing and tattooing, worn outrageous wigs, and squeezed themselves into constricting corsets, clothes, and shoes, all in slavish pursuit of their culture's ideal of beauty. Today, in every area of our lives—at work, while socializing, in the public eye—attractive people consistently get more attention than their acne-scarred, overweight, receding-chinned counterparts. What's worse, our culture is obsessed with celebrity, and the mass media multiply and magnify examples of human "perfection" every day. In such an environment, how tough is it to "just be yourself" and like it? (In a recent *People* magazine poll, an anemic 10 percent of women said they were satisfied with their bodies.) Add to all this an aging population with expectations (realistic or not) of prolonged youth. It's a marvel that everyone but two or three well-adjusted supermodels isn't wracked by feelings of inadequacy and low self-esteem.

The pressure is often felt most intensely in the workplace. Studies show that traditionally good-looking people are perceived as smarter and friendlier than others; they make more money, and are *five times* more likely to be hired. But this isn't a recent phenomenon: Even the ancient Greek philosopher Aristotle once said that "Beauty is better than all letters of recommendation." With the continuing influx of women and corporate downsizing making work environments more competitive than ever, there's increased pressure to look polished—*and* youthful. One of my patients, a thirty-eight-year-old publishing executive on whom I performed a neck and forehead lift, describes the pressure this way:

> *"In my profession I constantly interact with people, and I believe maintaining my looks gives me an edge. I'm not talking about being movie-star beautiful— who can be?—but I feel that appearing well put together, energetic, and youthful earns people's respect and attention, and ultimately gives me greater credibility. I am convinced looks make you money, so I think of surgery as an investment. Plastic surgery isn't just about beauty. It's about power."*

"Plastic surgery isn't just about beauty. It's about power." By allowing you to make subtle but important changes to your looks when and how *you* want, cosmetic surgery is a valuable, low-risk investment in your future health, happiness, and well-being.

ONE WOMAN GETS TO "YES"

Take Martha, for example. When the elegant sixty-three-year-old volunteer worker came in for an appointment, she told me she'd grown tired of striding confidently into a room, only to catch a glimpse of her reflection in a nearby mirror and feel that confidence disappear. "I just don't feel as tired and as old as I think I look," she said, despairingly.

I saw what Martha meant. While her voice projected energy and sharpness, she looked weary and her face was drawn. Yet she was reluctant to sign on for a cosmetic procedure, mostly for philosophical reasons. She felt that getting a face-lift was self-indulgent and a betrayal of her feminist beliefs. Her therapist, in fact, had counseled her *not* to seek a surgical remedy, urging her instead to deal with who she was and to accept her "limitations." Martha was too embarrassed even to discuss the issue with her grown children for fear that they would judge her harshly.

I pointed out to her that getting a face-lift, far from being a cop-out or an act of denial, can in fact be an effective, life-affirming way to embrace who you genuinely are. Although Martha's face did not reflect how she felt about herself, her negative feelings about how aging had diminished her spirit were absolutely valid. Should she have simply discounted her unhappiness? Of course not— and I think even her therapist would agree with that.

When Martha showed up two weeks later for a second consultation, she told me she'd come to see that wanting to look more attractive and vibrant was a worthy and respectable goal. "I'm confident in who I am, and my decision can't compromise that," she said. She had told her children about her plans, and was surprised at how supportive they were. Even I was astonished when she made the appointment for her surgery and asked for the works: forehead, eyes, neck, cheeks, lips! I won't say that Martha was anxiety-free: As the pre-surgery anesthesia was administered, she whispered to me, "I'm a liberal person by nature, but please be conservative!" Still, her feelings afterward spoke volumes: Martha was thrilled with the results, and she's confident she made the right move by taking control of her looks. And, happily, she's stopped avoiding mirrors.

THE LIGHT-BULB MOMENT

Like most of my patients, Martha didn't just one day decide to have cosmetic surgery, and I'm betting you didn't wake up this morning and, out of the blue, pick up this book. Probably for months, even years, a niggling voice in your head has been adding up all those "flaws" you just took stock of in the mirror. *Are those wrinkles?! . . . Since when have I had a double chin? . . . My butt is so big, I'd rather die than wear a bathing suit. . . . I wish my breasts weren't so droopy.*

After months or weeks or years of lowered self-esteem and mulling over the possibility of plastic surgery, *something*—an overheard comment, a death in the family, a milestone birthday, a divorce—will propel a person into my office demanding a change. A light goes on. "It was definitely a midlife crisis," says Toni, a fifty-one-year-old schoolteacher of her decision to have a face-lift, "but I'd already gotten my sports car in my thirties!" Here are just a few examples of such courageous decisions:

Light-Bulb Moment #1: The Photo Album

For Leslie, a fifty-nine-year-old attorney, her daughter's wedding was the impetus to have cosmetic surgery:

"My first daughter was married five years earlier. When I saw the photos, I was appalled. There I was over and over again: at the church, in the receiving line, and I looked tired and, well, *old*. I had always heard of people getting plastic surgery, but I thought it was something only movie stars did. Then a couple of years ago I went to a professional function where I talked with a woman I vaguely knew who was very open about telling me that she had just had some work done on her chin. For the first time, I thought, 'Gee, even people with average looks who aren't happy with their appearance can do something about it.'

"My younger daughter was planning a wedding that fall. Around Memorial Day I resolved to take care of the wrinkles on my face and neck before I was again forced to pose for all those family portraits. After looking together at the computer images of my face, the doctor and I decided we would do a rhinoplasty, eyelid lift, mini-forehead lift, and mini-face-lift. Although the recovery was somewhat difficult, by the fall I was feeling wonderful and looking great. I was more confident, and just plain happy to look so much younger.

"I could even tell that strangers reacted differently to me. You read articles about older women being invisible in our society. Maybe it was the way I carried myself—who knows? Whatever it was, I felt as if I was being noticed again, like I had been ten to twenty years ago."

Light-Bulb Moment #2: The Breakup

Alison was a long-term patient of mine. For years, she saw me for everything but surgery: glycolic peels, dermabrasion and laser for age spots, collagen injections—you name it.

"We were always talking about how, when I got to a certain point, I'd do something surgical," Alison, 42, recalls. "But I was happy with the smaller treatments I was getting, and figured I wouldn't need anything major until I was at least fifty.

"Then, suddenly, my marriage was in peril. I won't go into the details, but it was a blow to my ego. I was at the doctor to get fat injections in my lips, and brought up the subject of surgery. I was finally ready; I felt that getting a mini-lift would help me feel better and face the world anew. A few days later, I had the process. For the start of my recovery, I stayed in a hotel and had a round-the-clock nurse; I didn't want my husband to see me in such a state, especially considering the tension between us at the time. By the third week I was still a little swollen, but not too badly, and I felt I could finally face him. He was amazed, and frankly, impressed that I'd taken the initiative.

"Once you make up your mind to go through with surgery, it's really not a big deal," Alison continues. "I didn't dramatically change my appearance, nor do I look like some other person. I'm just a younger version of *myself*. I can't believe I'm approaching fifty, because I think—and people now tell me—I look like I'm in my late thirties."

Light-Bulb Moment #3: The Job Crisis

With increased pressure in today's shrinking workplace not only to perform, but also to look as if you have the energy, authority and competence to outperform everyone else, a growing number of professionals are turning to plastic surgery for a boost. Jim, a forty-six-year-old computer-industry executive, came to me not knowing exactly what remedy he was seeking:

"For months when I'd look in the mirror, my right eye appeared to be half closed. I kept thinking it was because I wasn't sleeping well, or maybe it was my sinuses. At work, you start to think that people are imagining that you've spent the previous night partying. Their reactions played tricks with me: I looked so unhealthy in the mirror, and suddenly I began to feel ill nearly all the time. I'm an older guy for the high-tech field; there are twenty-five-year-olds competing for the same jobs. I don't feel like a fogy, but making a good first impression can go a long way. I knew I had to do something if I wanted to continue to hold a position at this level.

"After my surgical consultation, I realized I wasn't sick. I was just getting older. In some people the skin around the eyes gets so slack with age it can affect their vision, and that was what was happening to me. So I signed up for upper and lower eyelid lifts on both eyes. I took a week off from work, and when I went back, nobody really said much. But the change was evident. No more offers for coffee or jokes about all-night drinking sprees. Now that I've decided to do something I've wanted to do for some time—to look for a new job—I am so glad I had the surgery."

Light-Bulb Moment #4: Facing Mortality

The death of a partner can also be a strong incentive to make a fresh start. Zelda, a therapist in her mid-sixties, told me:

"I have always prided myself on being a person who was committed to authenticity. When people talked about face-lifts and other types of plastic surgery, I argued vehemently about the need to accept aging and to feel comfortable with wrinkles and dark spots and sagging jowls. I believed that one should not succumb to the pressures of a popular culture that promotes youth and doesn't appreciate the positive qualities of 'seasoned seniors.'

"After becoming widowed in my late fifties, however, followed by a sudden mastectomy in my early sixties, I experienced strong feelings of sadness and loss. During a routine visit to remove age spots from my hands, the doctor broached the subject of performing plastic surgery in the form of a mini-face-lift, which, she gently suggested, would also serve as an 'ego lift.' I argued that I was not ready for a drastic change, and feared being labeled a self-indulgent narcissist. Most of all, I could not bear being seen as a different person—losing my 'self' through some kind of transformation. Several months later, after much thought and self-reflection, I made the leap of faith. For me, it was a courageous decision, and one that I've never once regretted.

"The procedure went smoothly. The discomfort and minimal pain were easily endured because the outcome was one I truly looked forward to. People said I looked rested and healthier than I had in years. I felt that I looked more like the person I was before these tragic events, and was delighted to feel that I had a new lease on life—a chance to care for my skin and not spend time lamenting the wrinkles that had begun to plague me. In these six years there has been some aging, but my inner sense of self is one of a youthful and energetic woman who is not immediately categorized by others as 'aged.' Movie-theater cashiers ask to see my Medicare card. This is a foolish delight, but it adds to my sense of self-esteem."

"I WANT TO, BUT . . ."

The stories above are just four examples of how life changes motivated patients to seize control of their looks—scenarios to which you yourself may relate.

Still, for all your enthusiasm, you probably also wrestle with doubts about the plastic surgery route. Join the club. It's the rare person who walks into my office *without* serious reservations about having cosmetic surgery. (I call it the "I Want to, but . . ." Syndrome.) And what sane person wouldn't have concerns? Although the media has publicized many of the amazing new surgical techniques available today, they've also perpetuated myths and sensationalized stories about botched procedures and unlicensed, scalpel-happy doctors.

We surgeons have to be more than just technicians; we've got to play psychologists too, listening to our patients' questions and helping them work through their anxieties and doubts. Every candidate for cosmetic surgery needs to reach her or his own comfort level, and for each person, the hurdle differs. One candidate fears the pain; another worries about how to explain, afterward, why she looks better than she has in years; another frets over the expense; still others fear that the result won't have the desired effect.

Let me share with you the most fundamental concerns my patients have voiced to me (and, of course, to themselves). They had to deal with these issues honestly and thoroughly before they could forge ahead with surgery.

THE QUESTIONS EVERY PATIENT ASKS . . . AND THE ANSWERS

Q: *"Am I just being vain?"*

A: Many people think that if you care about your appearance so much that you'd have plastic surgery done, then you're sinful or morally bankrupt. But why? Despite the increasing popularity of plastic surgery—according to the American Society for Aesthetic Plastic Surgery (ASAPS), 8.5 million cosmetic procedures were performed in the year 2001, an amazing 50 percent increase over the previous year, with baby boomers between thirty-five and fifty having the most work done—the skepticism and disapproval it can provoke still makes me marvel. This is especially so when so many of us, every single day, do all sorts of *other* things to make ourselves look better and feel younger. We diet. We color our hair. We whiten our teeth. We hire personal trainers. We spend billions yearly on over-the-counter skin-care products. We pop vitamins. We take hormone supplements. We get hair implants. We get facials. We take Viagra. Yet so many of us hesitate at the prospect of reaching these same goals with plastic surgery. Why?

Some believe it's "unnatural" to change one's body. Many feminists accuse women who opt for plastic surgery of caving in to male standards of beauty, or to the cult of youth. Other people argue that it's a hopeless gesture, external and superficial, that is only holding back the tides of the inevitable. But wanting to improve your appearance doesn't make you frivolous or superficial. In fact, as you have already heard from a few of my patients, there are manifestly *practical* reasons to maintain or improve your looks, from enhancing your earning power to staving off depression to actually improving the functioning of your body's largest organ—your skin. Is it vain to want to eliminate bags from under the eyes, especially when it can be done quickly, inexpensively, and with minimal recovery time? For men who've sported goatees since puberty, is it vain to want to fix that weak chin and stop hiding behind facial hair? For women embarrassed to wear fitted pants, is it vain to want to get rid of those saddlebags? For people chronically unhappy with their midsection, is it vain to want a waist that's more pleasing and youthful?

Perhaps. But if you're worried about being stigmatized, don't: In a recent study conducted by the American Association of Retired Persons (AARP), six of ten Americans over age fifty claim they'd have cosmetic surgery if they could, and more than three in four say they wouldn't be embarrassed if they had a procedure done and others found out about it.

Still, I understand how it's hard for many cosmetic surgery candidates to let go of the long-held belief that such a solution is narcissistic and undeserved. Sylvia, a fifty-year-old lawyer who comes to me regularly for microdermabrasion and light laser treatments, two skin-smoothing procedures, once confessed that she wanted to have her nose done. Yet the kind of person who gets a nose job could not possibly, in her view, be a modest, level-headed person who had achieved success through smarts, not looks—in other words, exactly the traits Sylvia saw in herself.

So what kicked her into gear? A colleague had recently confided in her that she'd had work done on her eyes and neck. The colleague looked terrific, and Sylvia couldn't believe the visible results, or the very idea of her having the procedure. "She's the last person on earth you would ever suspect would have something done!" Sylvia told me. "She's never fussed over her appearance, whether it's her clothes, hair, or makeup." Just seeing the results of a friend whom she respected, someone who was anything but a diva about her looks, gave Sylvia the courage to view things differently and schedule a nose job. Today Sylvia, the level-headed lawyer, has a smaller, less severe nose, and she says that the surgery has made a huge difference in how people look at her (literally!), as well as in how she sees herself.

Most patients who worry that they're being vain have legitimate body-image issues that they need to address. I hear the following all the time:

◆ "I feel as if my looks have aged, though I still feel young at heart."

◆ "I do anything to avoid revealing a physical flaw—like wearing baggy clothes or covering up a bathing suit, styling my hair a certain way, or refusing to wear open necks."

◆ "I've become increasingly self-conscious about my appearance."

◆ "I think my looks interfere with my being taken seriously at work, or may have held me back in my career."

◆ "At one time or another, someone—a spouse, friend, co-worker, even a stranger—has made negative comments about a physical flaw of mine, or referred to that feature in a way that undermined my confidence."

◆ "These days I flat-out refuse to undress in front of my partner or to make love with the lights on."

If even one of these statements sounds familiar, then toss out any notion that you're being frivolous. *When how you feel about your looks regularly affects your mood, confidence, relationships, or career, the problem is more than skin-deep. And if there's a solution that will help diminish or eliminate the problem, seeking that solution is hardly an act of vanity.* It's an act of practicality and common sense, and it's an important sign of your willingness to be pro-active about your own mental health and emotional well-being. In short, it's what you would do without hesitation about any other problem in your life.

Q: *"Will I look 'done'?"*

A: We can all recognize the hallmarks of the oft-nipped-and-tucked: the eyebrows arched in perpetual surprise, the pinched nose, the waxy skin, the taut neck, the wisps of hair carefully plastered in front of the earlobes to hide the telltale scars. This is a result of two things: an insistent patient with unrealistic dreams of youth, and a surgeon less interested in a natural-looking result than in fulfilling his or her patient's unrealistic dreams. My patient Martha, whose story I recounted earlier, said that one of the main factors that kept her from going ahead with surgery was the fear of looking "fake": "Of course we want to look better, but we also want to look like ourselves, not like a different person," she told me. "I can be enormously critical of other people, especially women of a certain age who have had their faces done to look like twenty-year-olds. I wanted to look a little fresher—less sad and drawn; I didn't want to look appalling."

If a procedure is performed well, friends and colleagues should not even suspect you've had work done; they'll just think you look great. I meet in advance with a patient to find a surgical strategy that addresses his or her concerns while preserving the face's innate harmony—a *very* important preparatory step. (For more on communicating with your doctor, see Chapter 4.) And fortunately, the technology has become so precise that we don't need to lift, or tuck, or suck as much as we used to in order to get dramatic—and *natural-looking*—results.

Q: *"How obvious will my scars be?"*

A: There's no such thing as totally scar-free surgery. But the scars from cosmetic surgery today are nothing like the big zippers of the past. Thanks to new techniques, it's unlikely that anyone will detect the telltale mark. Liposuction scars are a quarter-inch at most, the three tiny scars resulting from an endoscopic forehead lift are even smaller and are concealed by hair behind the forehead, and those from a breast augmentation can be nearly invisible when placed in the navel, in the armpit, or just below the nipple. One of my patients is a psychotherapist who feels it's imperative that none of her patients know she's had surgery (heaven forbid they should think she has "issues" of her own!). She has undergone two procedures, a face-lift and neck liposuction. Her patients all tell her how great she looks . . . and as far as she knows, they don't suspect a thing.

Q: *"How much pain will I feel?"*

A: Pain is the number-one anxiety patients have about going through with surgery. "I waited three years to have the procedure because I was terrified of how much it would hurt, especially during recovery," one breast-implant patient confessed recently. In the end, she characterized her post-operative discomfort as a "tweak" in her armpits and chest. Everyone has a different threshold, however, and the pain associated with each procedure can—and will—vary.

The surgery itself *should* be virtually painless. For almost every procedure, from the tiniest liposuction job to a whopping lower-body lift, you will have a local anesthetic and a mild intravenous sedative, which puts you into a twilight sleep—a state in which you don't entirely lose consciousness but are unaware of anything except perhaps some pressure in the area being treated. (Some doctors prefer general anesthesia for more extensive surgeries, such as a tummy tuck or thighplasty.) Afterward, I send patients home with prescription anti-inflammatories and painkillers, which they take for up to a week.

As a rule of thumb, the larger the incision, the tougher the recovery. More pain is to be expected when muscles and connective tissues—not just skin—are moved or tightened. A tummy tuck, where we make a hip-to-hip-incision and pull together the abdominal muscles underneath, will surely feel more painful in the days following the operation than will abdominal liposuction, which is performed through a quarter-inch hole beneath the navel and doesn't disturb the underlying muscle or tissue. Similarly, a neck lipectomy, which involves tightening the neck muscle, probably makes for a more difficult recovery than a simple neck liposuction.

Generally, the pain of the procedure itself isn't as bad or as memorable for patients as the recovery (there's more detail on this in Chapter 12). A patient may feel nauseated or groggy from the aftereffects of the anesthesia, while some report feeling itchy and uncomfortable for several days—"like my face was going to melt off," as one mini-lift patient described it. But I have never heard patients characterize the pain as something they couldn't handle without painkillers or anti-inflammatories. One of my patients has another theory: "Maybe it's like childbirth. You're so thrilled with the result, you just can't remember whether it hurt or not."

Q: *"How will I tell my friends and family—and whom should I tell?"*

A: Patients may be reluctant to tell a mate, child, or other relative or friend about wanting to have surgery because they fear those people will somehow see them as changed—that in making a physical alteration, they will also somehow have transformed their personality. I counsel my patients to assure the people they love that, yes, their character *will* be affected—happily so—because they'll feel better about their looks and more content with their lives. If you emphasize to your family and close friends how important it is for you to have their support, you're likely to get it.

Still, there are people in your life who may have a hard time accepting cosmetic surgery as a life-affirming choice. One of my patients told me that her husband threatened to leave her if she altered her face in any way. He wasn't being literal, she assured me, but this amounted to a significant *emotional* threat and was an indication of how adamantly he opposed the surgery. If you have an unsupportive spouse, family member, or friend, then only you can decide whether to go ahead with the procedure—and if you do, whether even to tell that person you're having something done. I repeat, this is a decision that *must be up to you.* Maybe that sounds deceptive, but I believe that in some situations—the exception, admittedly—keeping mum may be best. Five years ago, for instance, a young computer sales rep came to see me about correcting his weak chin. He told me he didn't want his girlfriend to know he was considering surgery, because she'd try to dissuade him. I thought, *What kind of relationship is this if he's not even going to tell her?* Just before the surgery was scheduled to happen, he spilled the beans to her. As predicted, she talked him out of it. What a shame, I thought, because he probably would have benefited from the surgery. More to the point, *he* wanted it, and in my judgment, it should have been his call, not hers.

QUOTE, UNQUOTE

" If you tell your friends and loved ones that you're planning to have a surgical procedure, they'll tell you they love you the way you are, that you don't need to change a thing. They are well intentioned, but you need to keep in mind that this is something you are doing for yourself, not for them. If *you* feel like you need surgery, then you probably do. I found it doesn't pay to listen to other people."

—Lynne, 57, former legal assistant

Sometimes a spouse or other loved one who opposes surgery is anxious about seeing you in pain. In that case, you just need to take a leap of faith and go through with it alone. Sparing a spouse from having to witness the recovery allows him or her to embrace the results—and your decision, if you so opt, to have another surgery down the road. "I didn't tell my husband until a couple of days before the procedure because he was very opposed to it, and because he can't stand to see me frail or ill," says Leslie, the fifty-nine-year-old attorney who had a mini-lift, along with a rhinoplasty and eyelid lift. "So I hired a nurse for the first two days and recovered in our city apartment while he stayed out at the house. It would have really thrown him to see me all black and blue." About six weeks after the operation, Leslie reported, her husband changed his tune: "When there was finally no trace of the surgery, my husband confided that although he had been against it from the beginning—he had thought I looked fine the way I was—he loved the results. A year later, when I had my neck done, he didn't protest." (This, by the way, is a not uncommon response once the work has actually been completed.)

When you're evaluating when and how to tell a spouse, relative, or close friend, keep in mind that, depending upon what type of surgery you have, you may need round-the-clock assistance during the first twenty-four hours afterward—to help you get around and get comfortable—and possibly for as many as three more days. (A lipo patient should feel quite steady one day post-op, whereas a tummy-tuck patient will have trouble standing up straight and generally fending for him- or herself for up to a week later.) A private nurse service can cost from $20 to $75 an hour, so patients whose spouses can't be supportive during this time may decide to widen their circle of confidantes to include a sister, daughter, or best friend.

Many patients wonder whether to tell their young children. Kids today are sophisticated. In fact, kids are the ones who often point out, "Mommy! What's that saggy thing under your chin?" Tactless but truthful, children are usually quite comfortable with the notion of doing something to "fix" a physical flaw. (Of course, you will want to refrain from explaining the operation in all its minute detail.) The key is to reassure them that you'll be exactly the same person after surgery that you were before. In my experience, grown children tend to be supportive. Here's what Elaine, who had a mini-face-lift and an endoscopic forehead and eyelid lift, had to say on the matter:

"You might be interested to know that I never told my children, a daughter and a son, thirty-one and thirty-three, about the full extent of my surgery. They are mother-oriented and, like most children, would feel it was not an appropriate thing for me to do. So I told my daughter that I was just going to have a little bit of work done around my eyes. That's all. We had dinner a month afterward and I was still a tad swollen, but she didn't ask me about it. Finally, as we were walking home, she turned to me and said, 'Whatever the doctor did, it looks wonderful.' That confirmed that I had made the right decision, and someday if she wants to ask me more about it, I'll be happy to tell her."

The bottom line: Each of us knows our loved ones best, so I try not to urge my patients one way or the other. If they need the support of my professional opinion, however, or a rationale that will reassure them and their friends and family, I consider it my responsibility to offer it.

Q: *"Isn't it unmasculine for a man to care about his appearance?"*

A: Men flock to gyms to pump iron and stare admiringly at their flexed abs and pecs. It's a small psychological leap from the gym to a plastic surgeon's office. For the last few years, the number of men wanting hair removal, skin resurfacing, and, more recently, neck liposuction and forehead lifts (among other procedures) has grown considerably. Startlingly, the number of cosmetic procedures performed on men increased 256 percent from 1997 to 2001, according to the ASAPS.

Today, men comprise 10 to 20 percent of my practice. After thousands of hours of conversations with hundreds of males, I can testify that they are no less concerned about their looks than women are. (A recent *New York* magazine cover story about male vanity and the increasing number of men seeking cosmetic treatments, corroborated this with the title, "Are Men the New Women?")

What's with the souped-up interest? At least half of it, in my opinion, has to do with career. A man who eliminates a paunch that months of pumping iron can't shake, or improves a weak chin that's been hiding under a beard, feels instantly recharged. His once-flagging confidence among co-workers, not to mention among peers and women who aren't colleagues, is replaced by self-esteem.

Q: *"How will I pay for surgery?"*

A: Plastic surgery is no longer just for movie stars trying to be forever young, or for rich dowagers with nothing better to do than lunch expensively, shop obsessively, and occupy themselves with repairing every physical flaw (real or imagined). While elective procedures aren't cheap, you don't need to sacrifice your life savings to afford them. Most people who have plastic surgery aren't rich: Two-thirds of cosmetic surgery patients have an annual household income of less than $50,000. They come from every walk of life, work hard for a living, and have decided that spending the money on how they look is justified.

Think of all the other ways we throw money at self-improvement. There's psychotherapy, for one: Just add up a year or two of getting shrunk and compare that cost to a $2,000 liposuction. It's probably a lot more! (And with no disrespect to my psychologist colleagues, which investment might have more immediate impact on your state of mind and self-esteem?) Add to that the amount you spent on clothes last year. Or the week you spent in the Caribbean lying in the sun, ruining your skin in the bargain. Do the math and you'll see that surgery is a reasonable expense for a long-lasting, effective remedy.

Fees, which vary by procedure, locale, and where the surgery is performed (hospital versus physician's office), range from hundreds to thousands of dollars and are typically paid up front (see chart below). Unless your problem is causing medical difficulties that surgery can relieve—as may be the case with breast reduction, rhinoplasty (nose job), or occasionally blepharoplasty (when vision is hampered by excess eyelid skin)—your insurance plan won't cover it.

Many of my patients use credit cards to cover the cost of their procedures; some use more than one credit card as well as a personal check. That's fine. The financial part of it shouldn't embarrass you. But before you decide to go through with a procedure, make sure you've made peace not only with your reservations and your significant others, but also with the expense involved. Your doctor's office manager can even help you devise a creative payment plan and steer you toward one of several lending institutions that has emerged to deal exclusively with payment for plastic surgery. These rates are generally comparable to those of most credit cards.)

The chart below represents the average cost for some of the most common procedures. The figures do not include the cost of anesthesia, medical tests, or prescriptions, which can run you hundreds more.

FEES FOR THE MOST POPULAR COSMETIC PROCEDURES

PROCEDURE	NATIONAL AVERAGE (in 2001)
Abdominoplasty (tummy tuck)	$4,477
Blepharoplasty (eyelid lift)	$2,510
Botox injection	$413
Breast augmentation	$3,257
Breast lift	$3,678
Breast reduction (women)	$5,183
Buttock lift	$4,616
Cheek implants	$2,376
Chemical peel	$831
Chin augmentation	$1,735
Collagen injection	$350
Dermabrasion	$1,367
Face-lift	$5,622
Fat injection	$1,065
Forehead lift	$2,779
Gynecomastia, treatment of	$2,894
Hair transplantation	$3,580
Laser hair removal	$423
Laser skin resurfacing (for treatment series)	$2,250
Laser treatment of leg veins	$427
Liposuction, traditional	$2,425
Liposuction, ultrasound-assisted	$2,551

PROCEDURE	NATIONAL AVERAGE (in 2001)
Lower body lift	$5,833
Otoplasty (ear surgery)	$2,589
Rhinoplasty (nose job)	$3,745
Thighplasty (thigh lift)	$4,078
Upper arm lift	$3,056

Reprinted with permission from the American Society for Aesthetic Plastic Surgery

As with any expense, consider clever ways to keep costs down. Fees can typically be reduced if you have more than one procedure simultaneously. For example, having laser resurfacing and a face-lift at the same time will almost certainly cost less than having the surgeries separately, since you'll save on anesthesia, prep time, and other overlapping fees. The surgeries needn't even be in the same area of the body; the same goes for, say, a nose job and breast augmentation done at once, or a chin implant and tummy liposuction.

QUOTE, UNQUOTE

"I'm not a rich woman, but I work out at a gym, buy high-end skin-care products, and I recently invested in a neck and forehead lift. The way I see it, I'd rather put my money into my body than into an expensive wardrobe that will be out of style in a couple of years."

—Beth, 54, publisher

When I was starting out in this field, it was common for women, many of whom didn't work in those days, to have to sheepishly ask their husbands for money to spend toward a cosmetic procedure. Now that so many women have achieved financial independence, *they* determine how much they are comfortable spending, and on what.

Q: *"Can you get addicted to plastic surgery?"*

A: Patients ask me this all the time. There are plastic surgery junkies who don't know when enough is enough. But it's the very rare person who allows herself to be turned into the Bride of Frankenstein. When someone looks like that, a bad surgeon must share the blame (either the same lousy one multiple times, or more than one irresponsible or unskilled surgeon). A good plastic surgeon simply doesn't let you get an excessive amount of work done.

But, no: Plastic surgery is not "addictive." And having one procedure doesn't necessarily mean you'll be returning for maintenance work either, though many patients refresh their look regularly with "quick fixes" such as Botox or collagen injections to eliminate wrinkles, or with a new surgical procedure every few years. That's because, quite often, when you start small and see what cosmetic surgery can do, you end up embracing its benefits. And I don't see anything wrong with that, so long as you're doing it for the right reasons: better health and looks, and greater control of your life.

Q: *"If I have medical issues, am I still a candidate?"*

A: If you've had cancer, a heart attack, or a history of chronic disease such as hypertension or diabetes, is it wise to put yourself through elective surgery? It depends. Surgery can be stressful, and any kind of stress can have a negative effect on your health. But since most contemporary plastic surgery doesn't require the use of general anesthesia, and is followed by a quick recovery, it is not likely to put you at any increased *medical* risk. Be sure to speak to your primary-care doctor about these issues beforehand. And of course be forthright with your plastic surgeon about any medical condition, since surgery may require temporarily stopping medications like blood thinners or aspirin (for more specifics, see Chapter 12).

Often, because of a patient's health, we may decide to perform a somewhat different procedure, though one that still yields similar results. Roger, an eighty-year-old actor with a chronic heart condition, came in for a facelift. After I spoke to his cardiologist, I decided instead to perform a necklift, a less invasive technique that would still give Roger the youthful tightening he was seeking on the lower half of his face. He was delighted with the effect—*and* the operation was shorter, with a quicker recovery and less stress.

Q: *"Is plastic surgery safe?"*

A: A big question, to which I can't give a blanket answer. With *any* invasive surgical procedure (including dental surgery) there is risk, from infection and bleeding to asymmetrical healing and nerve damage. And last decade's silicone implant scare has many women confused about which breast enhancement procedures are safe. But this is important: Plastic surgery—including breast and chin implants—*cannot* trigger an autoimmune infection or cause cancer. The substances we use in implants today are safe and FDA-approved.

Still, things can go wrong. I have had to revisit patients whose initial surgeries, by other physicians, left them looking disfigured; also, healing can be unpredictable, and a follow-up procedure is sometimes required to even out a ripply area or smooth a scar.

Later in the book I will discuss the safety of individual procedures. For now, the best way to protect yourself is to consult a board-certified plastic surgeon who is professionally bound to engage only in techniques that have been deemed safe—*after* rigorous testing. You can learn more about how to find a qualified specialist in Chapter 4.

There are no pat answers to any of these questions, but the first step to taking control of your looks is to ask them. The next step is to figure out which procedures are right for you and will help you achieve your personal best, so that you can find *your own* optimal beauty.

2

Personal Best: Getting the Result You Want

Once surgery is over, the first thing you want to hear friends, family, and co-workers say is "You look terrific!"—not "Who are you?" or, worse, "What have you *done* to yourself?" How do you get the result from cosmetic surgery that's best for you, and makes you happiest?

No two people have exactly the same idea of what's beautiful, nor is there one idea of physical beauty. Twenty years ago, when I started my practice, there was one nose, and only one nose, that plastic surgeons sculpted for a rhinoplasty: the "ski jump"—small, straight, and turned up at the end. Unfortunately for many of the women and men who had their noses fixed back then, this little proboscis looks ridiculous on their faces; clearly, their other features—long lips, say, or wide-set eyes—were originally organized around a more substantial central feature. Fixes for other body parts were also standardized—perky breasts, pouty lips, tightly pulled foreheads. There was little leeway for the patient's preference, and little consideration of how the newly enhanced feature would fit with the rest of the face or body.

Today, things are vastly improved. Surgical techniques allow for more variety in features; doctors are better listeners and take into account what will most satisfy a patient. No less profound than either of these two changes, there's also a far broader ethnic range of those seeking cosmetic surgery. My patients are black, white, Asian, Latino, and everything in between. They come from all over the world, including Europe, Israel, India, Japan, and South America. These racial and ethnic differences have influenced surgeons' approaches to beauty. For example, most non-Latina women yearn for smaller hips, but in the Latin culture, larger buttocks are often considered beautiful and sexy (think of Jennifer Lopez). I've had Middle Eastern patients looking to make their noses smaller, but—to retain both ethnicity and the integrity of the rest of their features—didn't want the WASP-y turned-up tip, or even to lose their nose's natural line.

WHAT SURGERY CAN AND CANNOT DO

The satisfaction my patients feel about what surgery can do for them, and what it ultimately *does* do for them, rests on their having realistic expectations. *If you come to a consultation with highly unrealistic hopes, the only outcome you can count on is your own disappointment.* No amount of lifting, tucking, or sucking will yield perfection, or make someone love you or stay with you.

Every so often, a patient comes to my office, holds up a picture of a celebrity or a supermodel, points to that person's nose or upper arms or stomach or legs, and says, "That's what I want." When that happens, I know their lofty hopes will be a hurdle for both of us. My first job is to bring such patients back to who they are. "Let's make your nose look better on *you*," I'll say, or "Let's improve your breasts so they are a better complement to your body." Imagining that plastic surgery can turn you into someone else is not a constructive way to start the journey toward self-improvement.

Counting on perfection is one red flag that I look for, so that I can manage expectations from the start. Here are other red flags for you—and a good surgeon—to watch for:

◆ *Red Flag #1: You're depressed.*

Lots of upsetting events impel patients to my office, including divorce, job loss, or the death of a loved one. When people go through an emotional crisis, getting plastic surgery can represent a positive, hopeful step. However, looking a little less wrinkly, or smoothing out the bump in your nose, will not make the painful sadness about other aspects of your life disappear. Breast implants are no substitute for psychotherapy.

When I interview prospective patients, I try to gauge their emotional state, and then adapt my recommendations accordingly. Still, I can't learn in an hour everything I might need to know about a patient. *You* must know whether you feel stable enough to make the right choice, especially if this is a time when you may not be quite "yourself."

◆ *Red Flag #2: You hate your body—all of it.*

Many patients tweak a half-dozen features, from head to toe—sometimes all at once, sometimes over time. There are few limits to what we can do surgically today. However, hating your whole body is a dangerous mindset from which to start. You won't have perspective on what elements of your appearance you want to change, and you won't be satisfied with the improvements you make.

◆ *Red Flag #3: You haven't tried nonsurgical options.*

Occasionally, I'll sense that a patient is rushing into surgery without first addressing the lifestyle changes that might bring about the desired improvement. For instance, if a very overweight man who has never tried to exercise or to improve his diet comes in wanting liposuction, I'm likely to postpone surgery until he develops healthier habits that will continue to support any surgical enhancements. (If I'm convinced that surgery would ultimately be in order regardless of the patient's lax habits, then I might do it anyway but also have him work with a trainer to get on a fat-burning, muscle-toning program.) Similarly, if a woman who still looks young wants to erase early stage wrinkles but has never followed a rigorous skin-care regimen, I'd start her on glycolic acids, topical antioxidants, and moisturizers. You can always progress to surgery, but the results you desire may be met just as well with nonsurgical interventions.

◆ *Red Flag #4: You're having surgery to please someone else.*

Cosmetic surgery isn't necessarily irreversible, but putting your body through any kind of surgery isn't to be taken lightly. If you make the change at the urging of a partner or friend or family member, then you're likely to regret it. I've seen too many women in their thirties come to me looking to increase the size of their nose—that's right, *increase*—because an overzealous parent convinced them to get a nose job in their teens, and now that their face and attitude have matured, the nose looks and feels wrong. And I've had women who come in with their husband to discuss breast enlargement, with *him* driving the discussion of size and shape. Sure, you want your partner to be happy. But whose breasts are they, anyway?

In the end, *you* must like the results. You're the one who has to endure the procedure, to recuperate, and to live with the change. And if the person you're making the change for is that picky about your appearance, the complaints won't stop with that lone cosmetic surgery fix.

◆ *Red Flag #5: You're back for a repeat performance.*

Many of my patients return to have another surgical procedure weeks or even years after a first one. That's perfectly acceptable: The body is a work in progress; a patient's looks continue to change as he or she ages; and besides, not everyone wants to (or can afford to) commit to having more than one surgery at a time. But if you've had plastic surgery on the same body part several times, or are slowly reworking every feature, head to toe, you may be suffering from a disease called Body Dysmorphic Disorder. BDD sufferers are preoccupied with real or imagined flaws in their appearance, and no number of surgeries will give these cosmetic surgery junkies satisfaction with the results. In the rare event that I think a patient is susceptible to this way of thinking, I will suggest the person get psychological support.

WHAT SURGERY *CAN* DO: REAL BEAUTY IS NATURAL BEAUTY

If what you're after is "natural" beauty—an appearance that makes your body or face look harmonious, healthy, and vital—then you're in luck. As a surgeon, my goal is to make each patient look his or her very best—*for the patient.* I can't make you look like Meg Ryan or Brad Pitt or Vanessa Williams. I *can* help you look and feel better than you did before, maybe better than you have in a long time.

What you are is what you are; cosmetic surgery just improves on what nature has given you.

Many of the potential patients who walk into my office don't know exactly what they want to change. Maybe they have a sense that they're looking older, or heavier, or that they walk around with a perpetual grimace. They may not even have noticed a problem until it was pointed out to them. A librarian in her forties came in recently and told me, "My kids keep telling me I look mad all the time." Only then did she zero in on the deep "scowl" lines between her eyes.

Often, too, a prospective patient may have only a general sense of dissatisfaction about his or her appearance. Not long ago I saw Cheryl, a forty-four-year-old actress. Her friend had recently undergone surgery and looked great, and Cheryl felt that she could also use a bit of rejuvenation. She complained about her eyes and crow's-feet, but I could see that the problem was her brow area: She wore a permanent frown that caused her eyes to droop, making her look older and more severe. While it's never my intention to insult a patient by pointing out a flaw she hasn't noticed, I gently indicated what, in my mind, the real problem was. Her shoulders sagged with relief. "You know, something about my forehead has always bothered me, but I'd never been able to isolate the problem," she said. So I did a forehead lift, which took ten years off her face, and the perma-scowl is gone.

I don't expect prospective patients to have complete self-awareness, but I encourage them to prepare for their first visit. If a patient that I meet for the first time throws up her hands and asks, "What do I need, Doc?," it's a problem—for her and for me. *You need to come in with your own ideas of what you want to change because, in the end, you're the one who needs to be pleased.*

Keep an Open Mind

You can guide the doctor by telling him or her why you're dissatisfied. Surgery is—or should be—a collaborative effort, not unlike how you might work with a decorator: You want to brighten a room, so you tell your decorator that you want an airier, more spacious feel. The decorator considers your suggestions about how to achieve that, but then uses his or her expertise and knowledge of color contrasts and the effects of light to realize your desired impression in the most harmonious manner. The point is the outcome rather than the means.

Narrow thinking and a presumptuous attitude won't get you positive results. I find, for instance, that some people come to me so well informed about various cosmetic procedures they've read about on the Internet or seen on TV that they'll insist on a plan of action that I think is inappropriate. Recently, Lance, a prominent artist in his fifties, came to me seeking a more youthful overall appearance. Because he also deals with aesthetics, he was quite certain that he wanted me to do a neck lift. I appreciated his analysis, but he was unaware of recent, maximally effective yet minimally invasive ways that surgery could accomplish the changes he sought. Together, we sat at the computer and looked at before-and-after pictures of other patients. Fortunately, he allowed me to work with him to devise a plan that satisfied both of us artistically—and medically. This included fat enhancement to his lips and nasolabial folds, an upper-eyelid lift, a neck lipoplasty, and chin augmentation. He quickly acknowledged that a plastic surgeon creates art in a different, *living* medium.

Occasionally I'll rule that a procedure is too risky, or an unhealthy solution to a problem. Once, a twenty-something Latina paralegal came to me about enlarging her buttocks. She wanted to increase their size by so much that she would need saline or silicone implants. Although this particular surgery has been done, it poses dangers: The patient would effectively be sitting on balloons, exposing herself to the risk of extrusion or puncture. It wasn't a chance I wanted to take. We ended up extracting fat from the abdomen and putting that into her buttocks. Her backside wasn't as large as she'd first hoped, but it was a safer, more organic solution.

Getting What You Want: The Means Versus the End

Given the many types of surgery available today (reviewed in Part Three) and the variables in people's appearance and health status, it's important to let your doctor help you decide which approach will work best for you. Sadly, there are doctors who *will* perform the surgery you want even when it's against their best judgment. Don't push it. It's against *your* best interest.

HOW MUCH TO DO?

It's common for patients to approach me with complaints about multiple physical flaws. They might be dissatisfied with their eyes, breasts, and stomach, or their neck and hips. So which makes more sense: to take care of everything at once, or to undergo each procedure separately? The answer depends of course on budget and one's comfort level with change, but also on the desired aesthetic outcome.

Like the old ditty says: "The hipbone's connected to the thighbone . . ." No body part is isolated. If I'm doing work on one area—the face, say, or the midsection—it often makes sense to correct more than one feature at a time, to preserve physical harmony. For example, I can lift the lower part of a man's face, but it may leave his eyes looking old and out of sync with his overall appearance. So I'll recommend doing both areas at once to ensure best results. Similarly, if I'm planning a breast reduction for a patient with a prominent lower abdomen, I will also discuss liposuction with her, because once her breasts are off her belly she may be shocked by what is suddenly visible.

If a patient is seriously weighing having two or more procedures, I might recommend having them done together to avoid the stress of a second recovery down the line (also, having two procedures at once is usually cheaper than having each done separately). Or, if I feel a patient will be receptive, I might suggest having an additional procedure "while they're under."

Doris, who came to me to tighten a sagging neck, came away with endoscopic forehead and eyelid lifts, too. As she recalls:

"While we were at the computer looking at surgical options for my chin, the doctor pointed out that the area around my eyes looked puffy and discolored. It was something I suppose I had noticed, but I was totally fixated on my neck. Lifting my forehead and the eye area could brighten the whole upper half of my face. I was just separated from my now ex-husband, and I thought it was the right time—it would be economical and I would have just one recovery period. So I said, Why not? In the end, I was so pleased I did it all. I felt refreshed and I looked good. It was a big boost at a vulnerable moment in my life."

Just as often, however, I do procedures individually. That may be purely, and justifiably, for financial reasons. If a patient has a budget of $10,000, that's not going to cover a breast reduction, liposuction, and nose job all at once. In that case, I'll help the patient determine which procedure she wants or needs most, and afterward help her plan a budget and timetable for the remaining fixes.

It's not just money that drives the all-at-once versus one-at-a-time quandary. Many patients are not emotionally prepared for multiple fixes at once, or to jump right into a major procedure. I call these people "tiptoers." They know they want *something* done, maybe even a few things, but they're nervous about committing to change. That's fine: Instead of going with an endoscopic forehead lift, for example, which can brighten and tighten the face from the nose up, I might start a tiptoer with microdermabrasion, a skin smoother, which requires no incision. Or a little Botox injection in the cheeks and forehead to provide a degree of wrinkle reduction until his or her reservations about having a face-lift are overcome.

Across the divide from the tiptoers are the "plungers"—patients who know what they want, and want it now. Plungers are the ones most likely to order up "the works." The advantages, of course, are that they undergo only one day of surgery; they have only one recovery period, which can simplify matters if time off from work is necessary; and the overall cost generally will be less than if the same work were spread over time.

CONFESSIONS OF A "TIPTOER"

"I first saw a plastic surgeon the year I turned sixty. I thought I would have a surgical procedure soon, but I got cold feet. My husband said he loved how I looked, and I just kept thinking, Why do it? Why put myself through the pain and expense? Over time, though, I really got comfortable with the idea. First we changed my skin-care regimen. Instead of slathering on moisturizer, which, the doctor claimed, only dried me out, I learned how to exfoliate with fruit acids and Retin-A, and I've never had dry skin since. We did some laser and microdermabrasion to get rid of blemishes. I followed this course for three years, all the while edging closer to smoothing out parts of my face, creating a less tired look. Finally the doctor gave me a little push, which was just what I needed. She said, 'If you don't do it now, what's the point of doing it at all?' She was right, and I put myself in her hands. Today, people tell me I look wonderful; others keep looking at me and asking if I've had a holiday or changed my hair. The results are subtle enough, however, that I don't think they can tell I've had surgery."

—Julia, 64, volunteer worker

CONFESSIONS OF A "PLUNGER"

"I'd always had a receding chin, and I wanted to get it built up. The doctor also suggested doing my eyes because the lids were falling; it was getting to the point where, in short order, my vision would be compromised. We went ahead and did the works. Five years later, I was having trouble with snoring. I went in for a recommendation, and discovered that I probably had a deviated septum. A nose job rectified the situation. Meanwhile, I mentioned that the underside of my neck had been getting kind of wattly, and we went ahead and fixed that, too."

—Sheldon, 68, retired sales executive

While I try to determine each patient's style and comfort level, I can't read minds. Each patient must be honest with me about his or her fears and concerns. Chances are you know yourself well enough to have some idea about which group you fall into (if either). If you're not sure, or you want extra guidance on how far to go, how fast, take the following quiz.

QUIZ: Are You a Tiptoer or a Plunger?

1 | When was the last time you radically changed your hairstyle?
(a) Recently—and often.
(b) Five years ago.
(c) I've worn my hair the same way since high school.

2 | In a moment of indulgence, you bought yourself a nice watch, even though it was clearly beyond your budget. Which applies?
(a) Whoa . . . I'd never do such a frivolous thing!
(b) I wear it with pleasure. What the heck?
(c) I keep it but feel guilty.

3 | How far in advance do you plan your vacations?
(a) I rarely plan ahead, preferring last-minute getaways.
(b) Two to three months.
(c) Six months or more.

4 | How do you make decisions?
(a) I go with my gut and can rarely be talked out of an opinion.
(b) I do a lot of hand-wringing and have a tough time making up my mind.
(c) I weigh the pros and cons before acting.

5 | Do you fall in love easily?
(a) Yes.
(b) No.

6 Look in your closet. How would you describe your wardrobe style?
(a) Conservative and monochromatic.
(b) Fashionable but consistent.
(c) Experimental and trendy.

Answers: Give yourself the corresponding points.

1. (a) 3 (b) 2 (c) 1   2. (a) 1 (b) 3 (c) 2   3. (a) 3 (b) 2 (c) 1
4. (a) 3 (b) 1 (c) 2   5. (a) 3 (b) 1   6. (a) 1 (b) 2 (c) 3

Now add up your points.

6–9: *You're a Tiptoer*. You don't need to be told to proceed with caution, because you always do. Have your doctor help you prioritize which procedures to consider now and which to save for the future. Start small—either with a nonsurgical fix to help you warm up to the idea of physical change, or with just one modest surgery. But stay open-minded. Your doctor may deem it necessary to make more than one fix at a time to maintain aesthetic harmony.

10–13: *You're a Middle-of-the-Roader*. More than half of all patients (not surprisingly) fall into this category. You listen to reason but are willing to go with the flow. It should be easy for you to work out with your doctor a sensible plan for your surgery or surgeries. You can always do more later.

14–18: *You're a Plunger*. You embrace change. You're confident in your ability to make the right decision. Just be sure, in your enthusiasm, that you adequately weigh the risks for the particular procedure(s) you're considering, and that you're willing to commit to the post-operative recovery process—which, because your body will be healing in several areas, will likely take longer. Finally, don't spend money you don't have. Some Plungers, fantasizing about the possibility of a life transformation, sign on for a total makeover. But going into debt to pay off the surgery isn't the way to make you feel better about yourself, even if you *look* better. Don't let yourself get carried away.

This quiz is just a guide to your level of intrepidness, and may be instructive in helping you figure out whether you'd be happier having lots of work done all at once or a little bit at a time. If possible, you should also talk with some people who've tiptoed into cosmetic surgery, as well as others who've plunged. Not only will they provide insight into the issues unique to each style of decision-making, but you may hear in one or another chronicler a sensibility very much like your own, which may further help you make your decision.

We've considered what kind of patient you might be. Now let's explore whether there's such a thing as the "right" time for surgery.

3

Why Now? Why Wait?: When to Start

A recent *New Yorker* cartoon shows two middle-aged women at lunch. With resignation, one sighs to the other, "It's too late for a nose job and too early for a face-lift."

Many people believe that plastic surgery, especially a face-lift or any kind of anti-aging procedure, must wait until they're in their sixties. Others, suspecting they've "missed the boat" on a particular type of surgery, never even seek youth-promoting alternatives. Still others fear that if they start down the road of cosmetic surgery too early, they're destined for a life of constant nipping and tucking.

Wrong, wrong, and wrong.

The best time for many cosmetic procedures, including endoscopic forehead surgery, facial contouring, or a neck lift, may be as early as forty. For other techniques, like lipo-suction, the prime age is even earlier, because skin that has just started to sag still has a wonderful ability to redrape—that is, to shrink and tighten, especially when underlying fat is removed. Over time, this redraping ability diminishes, so early intervention often helps a patient postpone or entirely avoid later surgery. Melissa, a patient of mine who at thirty-three elected to have liposuction on her waist and hips, describes how it helped her to take control of her looks:

"I believe in preventive medicine. So while I'm still relatively young, I felt I had to do something about a part of my body that has always given me grief—my love handles. I exercise every single day, and my weight has fluctuated, but I could never get rid of them. So I decided to have liposuction, and I love the results. It doesn't make me look drastically different—it's most obvious when I'm wearing a bathing suit—but I feel better about myself both when I'm wearing clothes and when I'm not. Plus, I don't have the frustration of go-nowhere workouts. Losing all that weight through lipo actually inspired me to lose even more on my own afterwards, and to keep it off."

To me, this is the ultimate fulfillment of cosmetic wellness, with successful surgery laying the groundwork for greater all-around health and well-being, as well as an enhanced ability to take control of one's life.

LIVE LONG, PROSPEROUSLY

A thirty-year-old American woman today can expect to live until she's seventy-five; two generations ago that figure was closer to sixty. A man, on average, will live to sixty-seven, versus fifty-eight forty years ago. What was considered "over-the-hill" way back when is not even approaching "the hill" today. Chances are you've made several changes to enjoy a longer, healthier life—taking vitamins, exercising, rethinking a stressful career, picking up a new hobby. (If you haven't, then get on it!) Why not live the next phase of your life looking as good as you feel?

60-Plus: You're Never Too Old to Look Better

If you don't act your age, why look it? (And even if you *do* act your age, you may not *want* to look it.) The fact is, you really can't be too old for plastic surgery, as long as you're in good health. But not every procedure is right for every age. For instance, I often see women in their fifties and sixties looking to rid themselves of the fat around their stomachs. One solution, called an abdominoplasty, is a procedure that removes fat and tightens the underlying muscles but requires a wide horizontal incision. So I'll often counsel women of this age to get liposuction, something we used to do only on much younger women. As with abdominoplasty, the success of lipo depends on the skin's ability to tighten (though not to the same extent). Is a woman in her sixties going to take off her clothes and look down at the same washboard abs as one in her twenties? No. But as long as she understands and accepts the limitations of a procedure on a body of her age, there's no reason not to do it. The same holds true for more modest procedures. Patients over the age of seventy—both men and women—come to me regularly for Botox or injectable fillers, microdermabrasion, and light-laser skin resurfacing. These procedures require no surgery or recovery time; they make the patients look better and consequently feel better about their appearance because they actually rejuvenate the skin.

From "Thirty-something" to Middle-Aged Spread

During the last ten years, baby boomers—that 800-pound gorilla of a demographic group born during the two decades following World War II—have moved squarely into midlife. The U.S. Census Bureau estimates that today nearly one in four Americans is fifty-five or older. Many in this group achieved considerable professional success early on, and, being generally fitter and healthier than their predecessors, are still far from retiring. Now, with generations X and Y nipping at their heels, and with the new economy forcing them to keep current with emerging technologies, boomers want help extending their stay at the top. That means looking well rested, vital, and more youthful.

Many boomers, notoriously in denial about aging, may not feel ready for cosmetic surgery and think of it as something to do when you apply for senior citizenship. In fact, now is just about the best time for them to have many of the procedures they've been considering. Since general health and lifestyle can dictate how well a person heals, baby boomers—who as a group smoke and drink less than did previous generations, while exercising and dieting more— are likely to enjoy more positive experiences with plastic surgery than their predecessors did. Their skin is likely to be healthy and resilient, and their ability to make a speedy, active recovery a near certainty. Moreover, as I regularly tell my patients who belong to this demographic, having even a light surgical procedure now may stave off *ever* having to go back to the operating table. It's that self-fulfilling act of cosmetic wellness: You take care of your skin, and the results—a more youthful look, perceptible improvements on the cellular level—jump-start a commitment to healthy living in other aspects of your life.

For many in their thirties or forties, a face-lift or other surgery may not yet be appropriate. But there are now so many other things we can do for those incipient crow's-feet, worry lines, or jowls. And these quick fixes are minimally invasive procedures—from light-laser treatment and microdermabrasion that smooth wrinkles to collagen injections that plump up loose and crepey areas—that don't even require an incision. (I describe them in more detail in Part Two.)

QUOTE, UNQUOTE

"My mother had a face-lift when she was sixty-five. I had mine a decade earlier because all of a sudden it hits you—you look *old*. It's like trying to define pornography: you can't really, but you know it when you see it. Well, I knew it when I saw it, and it wasn't pretty."

—Patricia, 53, public relations executive

The Young and the Restless

As more models, pop stars, and the MTV generation turn to cosmetic surgery for killer bodies, I've had a marked increase in the number of teens who come seeking treatment. Last year, according to the ASAPS, 15,000 reported cosmetic surgery procedures were performed on teens in the United States.

Now, I don't have a problem with a fourteen-year-old who wants to have laser hair removal. If her parents are willing to shell out for it, that's fine with me; not having to deal with razors and creams is more convenient for her. Moreover, if a teenager has what would be considered a physical deformity—a terribly oversized nose, ears that stick way out, or double-D breasts—then why should she have to go through puberty ashamed of her appearance or, in the case of very large breasts, physically hampered? I counsel young people the same way I would older patients: I review the most appropriate procedure for them, and make sure that they have realistic expectations and an understanding of their own role in—and commitment to—the healing process.

What happens when a fourteen-year-old comes in for liposuction or breast implants? It occurs all the time. While I may initially be skeptical about the reasons behind the desire for a smaller waist or bigger breasts, I consider each patient on a case-by-case basis. Some teens are not well suited for a cosmetic operation. Their bodies are still developing (bones continue to grow into the early twenties), and we must take extreme care not to interfere with Mother Nature prematurely. Also, the candidate may be mature physically but not emotionally, and thus unqualified to make a reasonable judgment about her looks. She may have been pushed into her decision by an overbearing parent or by peer pressure and the desire to fit in. Those Britney Spears videos, where the singer's breasts are pushed halfway up to her nose, don't help. What's more, a girl's notion of beauty is bound to change as she gets older, and as a teenager she may not truly realize that the decision she makes today is one she'll have to live with for many years. You'd think that her parents would grasp this fact, but you'd be surprised.

I do turn away inappropriate patients, especially those in their teens, or at least I'll suggest to them reasonable alternatives to surgery. Recently, for instance, a high school sophomore named Tara came in with her mother to complain about her heavy arms. Tara said that she'd exercised and dieted but that her arms remained bulky and lacked definition. Examining them, I saw what she meant, and if she'd come to me a decade later I would have refined their shape with liposuction. But at fifteen, a surgical remedy was unmerited. I explained to her that although she'd been using the Stairmaster and watching her weight, she was not doing exercises that target the arms, which yield terrific results when done correctly and regularly. I set her up with a personal trainer, who designed for her an upper-body strength-training program. After only one month of lifting, Tara began to see changes in tone and shape.

SOME TIMES OF LIFE ARE JUST NOT RIGHT

On occasion, I counsel patients to hold off before proceeding with surgery. I base the decision on how difficult it will be for the patient's lifestyle to accommodate major physiological change. Generally the patient is grateful for my caution, and in a few weeks or months we revisit the issue. Some especially complicating lifestyle factors that I look for:

◆ **Imminent Pregnancy.** Should you have major cosmetic surgery on your breasts or midsection if you're considering pregnancy? It depends. A woman in her early twenties seeking breast implants will likely not want to postpone the surgery until she decides to have a family, which may not be for several years. That's fine, of course. During pregnancy, your enhanced breasts will enlarge and engorge normally, just like breasts without implants. Typically, you will be able to breastfeed—especially if your implants are inserted under, rather than over, the pectoral (chest) muscles. When breastfeeding, however, some implant patients do report feeling more discomfort than non-implant patients.

Many women come to me after one or two babies, looking to have an abdominoplasty (tummy tuck); pregnancy has left them sagging and reluctant to get into a bathing suit, much less willing to get within fifty feet of a health-club locker room. They may not yet have decided whether to have another child, so surgery on that area is generally a low-risk option. If a patient plans on becoming pregnant within several months, I will counsel her to wait before going ahead with the procedure, since we don't want to stress the scar. Besides, given the havoc that pregnancy can wreak on the body, it's likely she'll decide she wants more surgery afterward.

◆ **Hectic lifestyle.** Among my patients are corporate executives, actors, and working mothers—some of the busiest people you could meet. I advise them that the small-incision, quick-recovery procedures available nowadays are compatible with their packed schedules and nonstop lifestyles. Nonetheless, a patient's life does have to accommodate post-operative recuperation, which can last anywhere from a few days to a few weeks, depending on the procedure. (Even after the incision itself heals, it is counterproductive to race around and divert the body's focus from making a full recovery.) An athlete who can't stop training to recuperate from a nose job, for instance, should wait until his or her competitive schedule eases up. Likewise, a businessperson who travels a lot or is unable to take off the several days needed for a face-lift to heal properly should wait for a vacation before taking the plunge.

◆ **Post-trauma.** Many people are desperate to make a positive change in their life after a bleak event, such as divorce, the death of a loved one, or a job loss. Often, a face-lift or tummy tuck can be just the thing to pull them out of their funk. However, depression clouds judgment. When I sense patients are feeling unusually negative about a life circumstance, I advise them to postpone surgery until they feel more in control of their emotions. They eventually may go through with the procedure, but I don't want them to do anything they will later regret, once the clouds have lifted.

Now that you have a better idea about the optimal time for surgery, let's consider how to find a doctor who can give you the results you're seeking.

4

The Right Partner: Choosing a Doctor

A few years ago, Meg, a twenty-seven-year-old associate professor who was both overweight and large-breasted, came to inquire about breast reduction. "Have you talked to anyone else about this?" I asked. The look of frustration, even anger, in Meg's eyes is something I won't forget. "Every doctor I visit says I have to lose weight before he'll help me," she said.

It's the same story I've heard from countless women with uncomfortably large breasts. And here's the interesting part: No matter how smart many of my male colleagues are, they don't seem to realize that a woman with double-D-sized breasts simply *can't exercise vigorously*. Even a good sports bra won't eliminate the pain and discomfort of jogging or doing Tae-Bo, to say nothing of the disincentive of being active with six pounds of mobile flesh hanging off your chest. After consulting with Meg, I scheduled her surgery, and I reduced her breast size to a C. Only then was she able to start a reasonable exercise program and lose weight.

Much has changed since I came into this profession in the 1970s, when the few women attending medical school were bluntly encouraged to be pediatricians or psychiatrists. I'll never forget my admissions interview. After exchanging niceties, the interviewer, a distinguished doctor, looked me square in the eye and said, "If I admit you, they'll think it's because you're an attractive woman." I couldn't believe it! This was Harvard? Before I even thought through my response, I shot back, "You're a good-looking man, doctor, and I can't imagine anyone thinks you got *your* job here because of it." Fortunately, he must not have taken my comment amiss, since I got a spot in the freshman class the next fall.

I believe that women have changed the way medicine is practiced, for the better. Women doctors, in general, have urged the rest of the medical profession to consider the doctor-patient relationship a partnership. Studies done in the mid- to late 1990s confirm that women physicians tend to be more attuned to patients' psychosocial needs and are better at communicating with patients than their male counterparts are. When you embark on the plastic surgery route, or opt for one procedure over another, that decision should be made jointly with your doctor. *As the surgeon, I'm the expert and must of course take a leadership position, but I make decisions with my patient, not for her.*

Take scarring, for example. Many of my predecessors, all male, once considered it acceptable—or at least not unacceptable—if a patient was left with a big scar. My personal inference was that scars matter less to men. A woman who got a face-lift in 1985 was typically left with big, clearly visible scars in her hairline and in front of her ears. What woman, when she gets undressed and looks in the mirror, or is out to dinner with a business client, doesn't care that the telltale signs of her surgery are obvious? A macho surgeon I knew once proclaimed, "If she wants her tummy tucked so she'll have a flat stomach, then the scar is the necessary trade-off."

I routinely discuss with my patients ways to do less of an operation. Are they willing to give up a little bit of the benefit of a full surgery if, in return, they're left with a smaller scar (not to mention enjoy a quicker recovery and lower cost)? Doesn't it seem like a bit of a Faustian bargain if, in improving your looks, the resulting scar makes you almost as self-conscious as your previous appearance did?

I am not suggesting that everyone, or at least every female patient, ought to have a female doctor. If nothing else, the suggestion is impractical: Only about one in twenty-five board-certified plastic surgeons in the United States are women. But your medical partner should be someone who can help you to understand the implications of the surgery from a more empathetic perspective, whether that doctor is female or male. Just as there are lots of things that doctors need to know to do their job well, there are a number of things that you, the prospective patient, need to know to choose your doctor wisely.

WHAT TO LOOK FOR IN A DOCTOR

It goes without saying that from your surgeon you want brilliance, understanding, resourcefulness, great training, the best hands and eyes in the business, and a calming manner. But you also need her or him to have professional qualifications. That may sound like a no-brainer, but the fact is, *anyone with a medical degree and a license to practice medicine can legally practice plastic surgery in the United States.* In other words, a podiatrist can perform a rhinoplasty; an OB-GYN can do liposuction. Spas, beauty centers, and even health clubs now offer procedures such as Botox injections and laser resurfacing, which are typically administered by non-M.D.s. They've proven to attract lots of business, and the profit margins are high.

No matter whom you pick, your doctor should have the proper certification and experience necessary to perform a given procedure. Since technology is constantly changing, such official certification helps to ensure that doctors keep up with the latest skills, and that they'll make the most of what they're learning. You should expect your doctor to be more than just aware of, but positively fluent in, such recent and dramatic advances as computer imaging, twilight sleep, endosocopy and other small-incision surgery techniques, liposuction, and "quick-fix" skin resurfacing techniques like microdermabrasion, light-laser treatments, and injections of collagen, fat, or Botox. Your doctor might take a course on a new laser treatment, for example. But the doctor will best comprehend the material if he or she has an extensive medical background in treating skin problems, watching how skin heals, and dealing with the complications that may arise.

To give another example, liposuction is a tricky procedure. In the hands of the untrained, it carries serious risks. If nerves are cut, this can result in permanent numbness. If too much fat is removed at one time, the patient may go into shock. When fat is removed unevenly, the skin surface may be left with unsightly ridges. Your confidence in both the doctor and the surgical result will be maximized when that doctor is skilled, experienced, and aware of current developments.

How do you know whether the doctor you're considering has years of experience or, instead, got her cosmetic surgery training at a weeklong crash course at a Las Vegas convention center? To keep from making an unwise choice, you should consider the following:

Board Certification and Creditable Associations: Six Degrees of Intimidation

Don't be impressed by the string of letters following a physician's name. While some of these acronyms represent legitimate educational degrees, others simply correspond to associations and societies that, in return for "certification," require little to join beyond the practitioner's office address and a checking account. *Be aware that there is no such medical specialty as "cosmetic surgery." In fact, if a doctor calls himself a cosmetic surgeon, you may have reason to be suspicious.*

Above all, your doctor should be board-certified. The most prestigious certification comes from the **American Board of Plastic Surgery** (**ABPS**), the official national examining board for professional plastic surgeons, whose members are qualified to perform reconstructive and plastic surgery, as well as aesthetic or cosmetic surgery. (To confirm that your doctor is board-certified, ask his or her receptionist, call the Philadelphia-based ABPS at 215-587-9322, or visit their website at www.abplsurg.org.) Doctors certified by the ABPS have earned a degree from an accredited medical school, completed at least three years of supervised general surgical training, served a two- to three-year residency training program in plastic surgery, and passed rigorous comprehensive written and oral exams.

That doesn't mean that only board-certified plastic surgeons are qualified to perform cosmetic procedures, or that a board-certified surgeon is always right for you. A dermatologist, for instance, might perform laser skin resurfacing, or an ophthalmologist might offer corrective eyelid surgery—procedures that they can be licensed to perform by taking a short course in the specialty. They may even be excellent at these procedures. But you should exercise caution. Will your doctor be able to handle complications during surgery or the healing process, should any arise? A board-certified plastic surgeon has had years of training in the handling and sculpting of skin tissue and its healing, and may be the doctor best equipped to handle the unexpected. Weigh the risks.

A few other associations and societies (as opposed to boards) are also highly creditable. Membership in one or more of them should be evidence that your surgeon shares its high professional standards. I belong to the **American Society for Aesthetic Plastic Surgery (ASAPS)**, which accepts only board-certified plastic surgeons who must submit several cases as evidence that they have done a requisite amount of aesthetic (or cosmetic) work. Another group with rigorous membership standards is the **American Society of Plastic Surgeons (ASPS)**, an educational foundation, which only doctors board-certified in plastic surgery may join.

You may notice that some surgeons have the initials **FACS** after their name. This stands for **Fellows of the American College of Surgeons**, an organization of M.D.s with all sorts of medical specialties, from cardiology to gastroenterology. The FACS requires its members to be board-certified in their specialty and to submit cases and letters of support, as well as to show affiliation with a hospital.

I belong to several other groups (the Laser Society, the Lipoplasty Society, and the Anti-Aging Society, to name three) because they produce informative newsletters and offer good opportunities for networking and continuing education. They don't, however, have a peer-reviewed membership policy.

You should also consider the accreditation of your doctor's hospital, even if your procedure is going to be performed in the surgeon's own facility. Moreover, if a physician has privileges to perform surgery at an accredited hospital, this signals that his or her performance and credentials are subjected to regular scrutiny. Without such affiliation, surgeons might be board-certified yet may have practiced for years without anyone keeping tabs on whether they have updated their methodologies or been the target of malpractice suits.

The Anesthesiologist

Finally, any surgical procedure will require an anesthesiologist (an anesthesiologist is an M.D., whereas an anesthetist is not). Make sure that he or she is certified by the **American Board of Anesthesiology (ABA)**. You may do so either by verifying the credentials with your doctor or, if you can find out your anesthesiologist's name in advance, by checking with the ABA (919-881-2570; www.abanes.org).

Know the New: Staying Up-to-Date

Most cutting-edge surgical techniques, such as endoscopy (in which a procedure is carried out under the skin using a miniature video camera), weren't taught when your doctor was in training. Not every plastic surgeon may choose to perform the latest procedures, and that's okay; there is no need to embrace every novelty that comes along. However, your surgeon should at least be *aware* of these procedures and able to discuss them with you knowledgeably. If not, that may suggest that the doctor isn't up on the latest available technologies for the surgeries she or he *does* perform. If you're contemplating a newer technique, find out whether your doctor uses it, and if not, why the doctor decided not to include it in his or her repertoire or seems to think it's not right for you. The doctor may have a sound reason, or may not have a clue. The latter should be your sign to continue in your search for a surgeon.

The Best Guide of All: Referrals

Finding a doctor you like and trust is a daunting task. How do you get a referral in which you have confidence? Today, with increased competition, many doctors—both good and bad—advertise on TV, radio, and even public transportation. Many more surgeons are quoted in national magazines or newspapers, or have marketed themselves on the Internet. Like a number of other physicians, I have my own informational website (www.drcopeland.com), and patients from all over have found me that way. But don't simply accept such exposure as credible testimony; it doesn't come close to carrying the weight of a credential or a recommendation from someone you trust. If you hear or see or read about a surgeon whose words or work interest you, you should do the same sleuthing you would to find out whether any surgeon is certified, affiliated with a hospital, and working out of an accredited facility. In short: Don't be impressed by a big name because it's a big name.

How about the dartboard method? That is, finding a name by consulting a plastic surgery member organization, or even by flipping through the Yellow Pages. That can be fine, too. The ASAPS offers a toll-free referral service (888-ASAPS11, which is 888-272-7711; or visit their website at www.surgery.org) providing names of board-certified plastic surgeons in your area. The ASPS also has a plastic surgery information/referral service: Call 888-475-2784, or try their website at www.plasticsurgery.org. Again, be sure to do your homework. No single source of information can be as good as multiple ones.

Should you ask your primary-care doctor or OB-GYN (or, for that matter, *any* doctor) for a referral? Sure—if you know your M.D. well, or if you have a friend who's a doctor and whose opinions you trust. Otherwise, be healthily skeptical. A doctor in another specialty may have no sense of a plastic surgeon's competency or, worse, may send you to a country-club buddy or someone with whom he or she is currying professional favor.

In my opinion, the best recommendation you can get comes from a friend who has had work done by a doctor he or she swears by. Most of my patients come to me via word-of-mouth. If you don't know anyone who can give you a firsthand testimonial about his or her experiences with the doctor you're considering, ask the surgeon whether you can talk to some former patients.

"FACE-LIFTS—GOING, GOING . . . GONE!"

Bidding for surgery? That's the worrisome new trend practiced on several websites created to help prospective patients find the least expensive fees around. On one site, for instance, member-surgeons have seventy-two hours to bid against each other for the job. At another, consumers state how much they're willing to pay for a procedure, and the site makes referrals to surgeons who will do it at that price. But too often, cheapness doesn't coincide with quality, and typically these sites do not accept liability for botched surgeries (that should be a red flag right there). My advice is to indulge your inner bargain hunter on eBay. When choosing a doctor, rely on intelligence, experience, thoroughness, and caution, not impulse. Do you really want to tell people, "I picked my surgeon because he bid the lowest"?

THE CONSULTATION

You don't just want a good doctor, you want a *partner*: someone who listens to your concerns, gives weight to your fears, and fills you with reassurance about the decision you are making. A partner should have a personal style that makes you feel comfort and trust. Some surgeons are highly skilled technicians with the bedside manner of Quasimodo. Whenever I myself see a doctor, it's important to me that he or she listen to all my questions and give me patient, thoughtful answers. I also want to know that a doctor will be there for me not just during a procedure, but for the recovery and healing process, too. A doctor who hustles you in and out of a consultation in fifteen minutes may be too busy to focus on your needs, or may delegate a great deal of responsibility to a nurse or other technician. Again, that's not necessarily bad. But I would prefer that *my* surgeon spend roughly a full hour with me, attentively answering my questions and offering insight and reassurance. This, at least, is what I try to do for my patients.

A good partner also includes you in decision-making about what procedure or set of procedures is right for you. It's easy for me to say that I think you need a mini-lift or a chin implant; part of my job is to have a practiced eye for spotting asymmetry and disfiguring flaws. But surgery isn't *always* the answer—or not right away, at any rate.

For instance, when Patricia came to me a couple of years ago, she wanted to do something about her sagging neck. "One doctor told me to get my picture taken and to show up on the appointed day," she said. "Another told me to lose weight and then he'd cut the excess skin out. It was as if they didn't want me as their patient." By the time she found me, Patricia was extremely dispirited. I could see that a mini-lift would remedy the jowly look she had developed, but first I wanted to put her on a skin-care program and perform microdermabrasion to get rid of her acne scars. Without doing so, the results of her face-lift might have been compromised.

Cosmetic surgery is nothing if not personal, and it represents a dramatic "taking-charge." *By laying out your options, rather than just arbitrating what she or he wants to do, a surgeon allows you to be the one who decides it's time for a change, and what kind of change you want to make.* You, and no one else, will have to deal with the recovery, and live with the results.

The right partnership can create a long-lasting bond. Some of my patients have been with me for more than ten years, and come back regularly between surgeries (if they have more than one) for "tune-ups," from laser treatments to advice on skin creams. "These last few years leading up to my face surgery were a process," recalls Julia. "First we spent three years giving my skin a nice glow with microdermabrasion and a skin-care regimen. Then I had my mini-lift. Now I go in periodically for Botox injections and laser treatment. I told the doctor I'd likely be with her forever."

The First Visit

What should be accomplished at the first consultation? You should learn about your doctor's manner, credentials, and recommendation for a course of action. Many patients, anxious about their first time, treat a consultation like a job interview—as if they have to pass some sort of test. True, the doctor is asking a lot of questions; as I sit across the desk, I evaluate what procedure seems appropriate for a patient, whether that person's expectations are realistic, and how his or her body will likely react during and after surgery. But the consultation is your time to grill the doctor, so be an active participant.

When prospective patients arrive for a consultation, I have them fill out an "intake"—an application that asks for name, basic medical history, and why they've come. This information, which my assistant shows me minutes before an appointment, gives me a basic sense of a person's complaint and background. I then open the interview by asking what brought the patient to my office, and then have the person elaborate on what part or parts of the body and/or face concern him or her most, and why. There are no right or wrong answers. Mostly, I listen for cues that tell me how enthusiastic or nervous a person is, and whether the his or her expectations are realistic.

" I decided with a friend that we would get breast implants together. We came up with a bunch of names from the Net, and visited several doctors in the New York area and as far away as Philadelphia. One doctor scared us both away. We wanted to get bigger, but his idea of big was *huge*. Other doctors said, 'We can do this for you tomorrow. Just sign on the dotted line.' I needed time, and kept looking until I found a doctor who explained the whole procedure, and then told me to come back when I was ready. I was so glad to have found the right match, I didn't even mull over the decision. I scheduled surgery right away."

—Chantal, 27, actress

Ask, Ask, Ask

Everyone's first impulse is to ask, "What do *you* think I need?" This is a perfectly valid question, and one that I'm happy to answer after I hear what a patient's concerns are. This is, if anything, a matter of tact. If someone tells me she is concerned about her eyes and forehead, and the first thing I notice is her enormous breasts, I'm not going to recommend she have a reduction. Beauty is in the eye of the beholder, and I don't want to draw attention to a "flaw" if it isn't making the other person unhappy. If, however, a patient feels his face looks aged but can't put his finger on what feature is the culprit, it is my job to point out that a forehead lift and eye job would give him the more alert, youthful look he seeks.

Many patients come to the consultation with a checklist of questions. Usually I ask them to hold off on asking them until the end of our meeting, since I will address many of them during our discussion. Not all prospective patients get their questions answered, either because they don't know what the questions are or are hesitant to ask them, or because they feel the doctor doesn't have the time for so many queries. That's not acceptable. There are a minimum number of facts you should have drawn out by the time you leave a first consultation.

Questions to Ask Your Doctor at the First Consultation

✔ Which technique(s) do you recommend to solve my problem?

✔ What are the risks and advantages of each alternative?

✔ How often do you perform this type of procedure?

✔ How long can I expect the effect to last?

✔ Where will the surgery be done?

✔ Will my medical history interfere with the procedure you recommend?

✔ What should I know about the side effects of one procedure versus another?

✔ Are there medical or lab tests I'll need to undergo before surgery?

✔ What kind of anesthesia will you use?

✔ What does the procedure involve, and where will the incisions be made?

✔ How long will the surgery take?

✔ What is the pain like?

✔ How involved are you after surgery?

✔ How long will the recovery take? What does it entail?

✔ Will I need someone to take me home? Someone to stay with me? If so, for how long?

✔ Are there potential reactions or side effects that I should expect?

✔ How common are complications with this procedure?

✔ When can I return to work? To exercising?

✔ How soon after the procedure should I come in for a visit? How many post-op visits are there? Are they all covered by the initial fee?

✔ Is there anything I'll have to do differently after the procedure?

✔ When will I be able to see the results?

✔ What are your fees and payment terms?

Note: No doctor trumpets the mishaps that he or she has experienced. But honest doctors, in answering the relevant questions, will tell you frankly about potential risks and any rare complications. If all you hear is good news and unmitigated success, then you have to trust your gut to tell you if the surgeon is being straight with you.

The Proof Is in the Picture

I firmly believe that photography should play a role in any consultation. We plastic surgeons rely heavily on taking and interpreting pictures. In residency, we're trained to use a camera to document patients before and after procedures so that we can keep accurate medical records. Pictures also aid us in having a thorough, successful consultation—and are handy during surgery. In the operating room, I keep a "before" picture of the patient right next to me. I refer to it, ensuring that I'm doing exactly what we agreed upon.

Today, computer imaging software allows us to photograph you and then immediately manipulate your features onscreen, so that you have an idea of a procedure's "aftereffect." Although you won't come out looking exactly as you do onscreen, the resulting image makes the results concrete and exciting, and helps with decision making.

Not every doctor uses computer imaging. But during a consultation, the doctor should at least show you images reflecting the results of the procedure you're considering, rather than speaking about them abstractly. Seeing photographs can also give you a sense of a surgeon's aesthetics. You may find that all of a surgeon's rhinoplasty patients have the same exact little Barbie-doll nose, or that the forehead-lift patients all look severely pulled. More likely, though, the images will just help you better visualize the procedure.

Second Helpings

Patients often wonder about these two questions (though rarely ask the first): Should I get a second opinion? And, should I have a second consultation with the doctor I choose?

To each, I say—maybe. If you feel secure with and confident about a doctor you've "interviewed," and you like what you hear about him or her from others, then go with your instinct. On the other hand, if you're uncertain about whether the surgeon is best for you, or whether the procedure he or she has recommended is ideal, then obviously you should keep looking. The next doctor you see may have a very different idea of how to achieve your desired result.

As for second consultations: I'll sometimes see a patient again, free of charge, if I sense that he or she is a "tiptoer," and is especially nervous about a procedure, or if we haven't completely agreed on a course of action. Every doctor has his or her own approach, and many make a second consultation routine before proceeding with surgery.

The bottom line is that you should *never* proceed with surgery until you are ready. Some of my patients have developed cold feet in the days leading up to the procedure, and sometimes we've postponed the date until they fully believed they were making the right decision.

SHOULD YOU TRUST THE INTERNET?

A couple of years ago, a rumor circulated on the Internet that plastic surgeons routinely and secretly injected fat from one patient into another, without notifying them. Although the Net has become an invaluable source of information, there's also a great deal of online info that's far-out, alarmist, and just plain wrong.

Surgery candidates often find it useful to talk in a chat room or on bulletin boards with those who are also contemplating a procedure or who have already undergone surgery. However, you should temper your response to a lot of the medical information you find online. Misleading advice is propagated by people who call themselves "experts," who hang out a virtual shingle but have no formal training or technical knowledge of what they're talking about. And the Net has become a forum for those enraged about surgeries gone wrong, which may terrify candidates into thinking that a procedure is categorically unsafe.

INFORMATIVE AND TRUSTWORTHY WEBSITES

I find the first two sites below to be excellent information sources from well-established associations; the second two are from private companies that offer fun and useful services.

◆ www.plasticsurgery.org: The official site for the American Society of Plastic Surgery (ASPS). It provides profiles of doctors and offers referrals in your area. It includes FAQs (frequently asked questions), recent FDA concerns and approvals, the safety record of certain procedures, and a detailed explanation of each. You'll also find intriguing statistics and costs.

◆ www.surgery.org: The official site of the American Society for Aesthetic Plastic Surgery (ASAPS) can help you find a board-certified plastic surgeon near you. It includes write-ups on the latest trends, safety concerns and procedures, and a gallery of before-and-after photos for many procedures.

◆ www.implantinfo.com, www.liposite.com, www.faceforum.com: These lively patient-to-patient Websites offer an opportunity to share information on procedures, price, and doctor selection with others who have undergone plastic surgery.

◆ www.ienhance.com: This site helps you locate a specialist close by, features a photo gallery of before-and-after pictures, and includes detailed explanations of hundreds of procedures. It also features first-person testimonials such as "My Experience with Retin-A." See the Patient Financing section for a discussion of costs and affordability.

Now that you've completed Part One of this book and know what qualities and qualifications to look for in a surgeon, you've made the first move toward taking control of your looks. Next, let's get specific about actually improving your appearance—and the way you feel about yourself—in ways you wouldn't have imagined possible.

For those who aren't yet ready to take that big surgical step, or who want to lay the groundwork for surgery with smoother, better-looking skin, I will first talk about the myriad *nonsurgical* cosmetic interventions you can, and often *should*, take first—both those pursued under a doctor's supervision and those pursued on your own. These therapies—some of them cutting-edge technologies, others tried-and-true methods—are a quick, easy way to make a lasting investment in your skin and your future cosmetic wellness.

PART TWO

Skin Savers and Quick Fixes

5

The First Step: Caring for Your Skin . . . the Right Way

Your skin is you. More than any other feature of the body, it announces, "I'm young and healthy," or "I'm letting myself go," or "I smoke like a chimney," or "I still haven't figured out that baking in the sun is harmful."

Our skin is a living, breathing road map of the lives we lead and have led, right out there for all to read. Fortunately, you can chart your own course for the future. In the last decade we've made amazing advances in the science of the skin. Because we now understand the mechanism by which it matures, we can start to reverse the skin's aging process and nurture it to become healthier and younger.

Until ten years ago, I had trouble convincing patients to follow any kind of skin-care regimen. As a plastic surgery resident, I encouraged my patients to use exfoliants and moisturizers; a trained chemist, I am particularly cognizant of the active properties of certain molecules in topical acids and vitamins, and their potentially transformative effects on the skin. For the most part, however, my colleagues at the hospital weren't interested in pre- and post-surgical skin care—they did what they did in the operating room, and didn't see their patients very far into the recovery process. Still, I urged my own patients to stay aware of the big picture: We can nip and tuck you from every angle, but if your skin is discolored, overly dry, or damaged, you won't see the beautiful result you were hoping for, no matter how much surgery you undergo.

An example: Last week, a woman in her fifties came into my office. She'd had her eyes done, as well as her nose, cheeks, and forehead—the works (though by someone else). Clearly, she'd spent considerable money and time on a younger appearance, but she looked *old* because her skin was in terrible shape. Around her mouth and forehead were wrinkles and blotches from sunbathing and who knows what other careless habits. What's the point of all that surgery if you don't take basic steps to maintain the health and vitality of your skin?

IS THAT A *WRINKLE*?!

Healthy skin constantly sheds and regenerates itself. But as we age, our skin becomes sluggish. It doesn't "turn over" and rid itself of dead cells as quickly. Instead, the cells pile up, causing wrinkles, discoloration, and general skin laxity. The collagen—tiny stacked fibers that control the skin's elasticity—loses its alignment, and its layers become more loosely stacked.

How precipitous is the downturn in resiliency? That depends in part on heredity (which influences skin color), musculature, bone structure, and hormone levels (sufficient estrogen is connected to healthy, glowing skin). But there are several environmental, and often preventable, ways that we speed our skin's descent into old age.

◆ **Sun exposure**. Simply put, sun is the single most prominent factor in the aging of skin. Solar radiation doesn't just alter the skin's pigmentation; it penetrates deeply, disrupting and weakening the skin's collagen and elastin (another layer that holds skin together), thereby affecting the way cells turn over. Sun also causes outbreaks of broken blood vessels and triggers the release of free radicals—destructive molecules that change cells' DNA and can lead to the manufacture of pre-cancerous changes in skin.

◆ **Pollution and smoking**. Environmental and tobacco-generated pollutants also contribute to the release of free radicals, interfering with the skin's ability to reproduce the way it should. Smoking in particular reduces the blood supply—and hence oxygen supply—to the skin, leaving it ravaged and aged.

◆ **Dieting**. Chronic (also known as "yo-yo") dieters inflict repeated damage on their skin. Gaining weight causes skin to stretch, compromising its elasticity, and losing pounds leaves it saggy and sallow, resulting in more prominent wrinkles.

REVERSAL OF FORTUNE: REJUVENATING YOUR SKIN

The skin is an organ (the body's largest, in fact). Just as we exercise to keep our hearts healthy, we must take certain measures to boost our skin's health. Skin acts, first and foremost, as a barrier to bacteria. Healthy skin is moist and supple; when it gets dry and cracked, it becomes prone to infection. Second, skin that's not encouraged to turn over regularly is at greater risk for complications, from discoloration to pre-cancerous changes. *So taking care of your skin isn't just about looking good; it's also smart and healthy, part of an everyday approach to cosmetic wellness.*

There are four phases to maintaining healthy skin: cleansing, exfoliating, moisturizing, and sun protection. Now, I don't seriously expect everyone to have the time to address every single phase regularly. Some people, for example, are vigilant about brushing their teeth, flossing, and using a Water Pik several times a day, while others can barely get themselves to brush before they go to sleep. That's normal and human. So rather than assign a time-pressed patient a Draconian regimen that won't be sustained, I design a quick routine to suit a busy lifestyle. Once patients see for themselves that their skin can look demonstrably healthier in as little as two weeks, they're more likely to embrace a consistent program and find creative ways to fit it comfortably into their life. After considerable practice, I've become very good at applying up to six skin-care products each morning between blow-drying my hair, making coffee, and getting dressed.

Here's more on the four phases, and why they are all necessary:

1. Cleansing

Why is it important to keep your skin clean? For the same reason that you brush your teeth every day. The surface of your skin is inhabited by millions of bacteria. Inevitably, some of those bacteria find cracks or dry patches, get under the surface, cause infection, and weaken skin integrity. Regular cleansing helps to eliminate these insidious germs.

But not just any kind of cleansing will do: When patients first visit with me, many if not most of them are soap users. But soap can change the pH, or acidity level, of the skin, causing it to become irritated and dried out. We know this from studies on cells grown inside test tubes: When the pH is altered, development is slowed. I encourage soap users to ditch their standard bar in favor of a gentler cleanser, one with no perfume and fewer additives. These cleansers will remove dirt from the skin while maintaining the proper environment for cell renewal. I also encourage patients to use a toner after cleansing—not the type of de-greasing, astringent toner in widespread use a decade ago, which stripped the skin of essential oils, but an alcohol-free toner that helps maintain the skin's pH balance.

2. Exfoliation and Cell Renewal

As we age, the skin's ability to regenerate slows. Plastic surgeons have long known that by removing the top layer of skin, we can speed the turnover process. We observed this phenomenon by doing reconstructive work on burn victims: Although deep burns carried a big risk of scarring, superficial burns—where just the top layer of skin had come off—caused the skin to heal without wrinkles, and at times looked even better than it had before the burn!

Chemical Peels
Building on what we knew about the biology of superficial burns, we eventually discovered that certain acids, when used on the skin, would penetrate and remove the top layer, sending a signal to the cells in the layers below to pro-

duce more cells. What a revelation! Over the years, we've developed several types of chemical exfoliants for this purpose, which are left on the skin for a short time and then removed. In high concentrations, chemical peels are usually performed in a doctor's office. Lighter peel formulas available over the counter contain some of the same chemicals as prescription peels, but are not nearly as effective.

- **Phenol** is the strongest of the solutions used for peeling. Developed in the 1950s, it penetrates so deeply that the skin peels abundantly for days after treatment. Phenol carries a risk of scarring and permanent hypopigmentation, or skin whitening, so it's never used on darker skin tones. Today, phenol may still be used when a very deep peel is desired, but most doctors choose lighter acids for greater control.

- **Trichloracetic acid (TCA)** is gentler than phenol, and gives a medium-depth peel. As with phenol, however, TCA can leave the face so raw and red after a treatment, and make the skin flake so profusely, that it may take two weeks before a patient feels comfortable even going outside.

- **Alpha- and beta-hydroxy acids.** Developed in the 1990s, alpha-hydroxy (AHA) and beta-hydroxy (BHA) acids, derived from fruit, plants, milk, and other natural sources, have revolutionized the peeling business. (Glycolic acid, which comes from sugar cane, is one of the most popular types of AHAs.) These acids have been in use for a long time: Cleopatra rubbed milk and lemon juice on her skin, a form of acid exfoliation. Because these acids are produced in lighter concentrations than phenol or TCA, they produce a gentler peel. They are very effective (and safe!) for regular use, jump-starting cell turnover and tightening the skin. After these acids are applied, the skin may be a little red, and moderate sloughing may occur a few days later. However, you won't experience anything like the "paint-chip" flaking that results from using phenol or TCA. AHAs and BHAs have thus gained currency as reliable quick fixes or "lunchtime" peels that may be done frequently in the doctor's office or at home.

Not if you can help it. Rags, loofahs, and brushes are loaded with bacteria. When you scrub the skin, it causes microscopic cracks to develop, allowing bacteria to get in and setting you up for infection. Instead, rinse with water and use a gentle cleanser, rubbing it in with your fingertips. Follow that with a topical exfoliant to slough off the top layer of dead skin. I also recommend abrasive scrubs, which help skin exfoliate, and clay masks, which act like a poultice, drawing out oil. Leave the rags for cleaning the house!

Other Topical Treatments

◆ **Retin-A.** The development of Retin-A (the trade name for the chemical tretinoin) in the 1960s represents a great stride. A type of vitamin A originally formulated to treat acne, Retin-A was found to deliver great cosmetic results on wrinkles, too, by helping the skin to regenerate. It works differently from acids, however, which stimulate new cell growth indirectly by removing the top layer of skin. Rather, Retin-A goes directly to cells, sending them a signal to generate. It also increases blood supply to the skin and helps the alignment of collagen. The downside? The risk of irritation and increased blood vessel formation. The very popular Renova, a brand that appeared in the mid-1990s, is minimally irritating, but today its use has mostly been overshadowed by acid peels.

Yes, but it's not advisable. Tretinoin, the active ingredient in Retin-A, is not only inactivated by sunlight; it also tends to thin the stratum corneum, the outermost layer of the skin, causing greater vulnerability to sun damage. So if you absolutely must be in the sun all day, wear a hat, use a full-spectrum, high-SPF sunblock, and apply the Retin-A at night.

◆ **Antioxidants.** I like my patients to follow an acid treatment with a topical antioxidant vitamin, such as C or E, which fights oxidants, or "free radicals"—the unstable molecules caused by exposure to sun and pollution that age the skin. We've long known that vitamins are important for healing: Sailors who for weeks went without fresh produce, and hence vitamin C, would get scurvy and suffer connective tissue problems. More recently, we've discovered that if you put vitamin C on the skin, it improves the alignment of collagen and triggers skin regrowth.

3. Moisturizing

Children's skin naturally stays soft and supple. With age, skin is no longer able to replenish its own moisture. Drinking eight glasses of water a day, while good for the complexion, isn't enough to keep skin youthful and hydrated; a penetrating moisturizer is needed to deliver water to the skin's cells, keeping them full and balanced, and to seal that moisture in. Moisturizers that contain alcohol will contribute to dryness; those that contain too much oil can clog pores and create dirt buildup.

URGENT QUESTION:

DO OVER-THE-COUNTER ANTI-AGING PRODUCTS WORK?

They certainly won't hurt you, but a $100 jar of "revitalizing serum" is unlikely to contain enough of any active ingredient to effect much of a change in your skin. For instance, the concentration of glycolic acid in the formula a doctor dispenses is typically 8 to 20 percent, whereas the percentage in a store-bought product is usually less than 5 percent. For vitamin C and other antioxidants, the over-the-counter (OTC) percentage is even lower.

To help their patients navigate the confusing (and expensive) plethora of products out there, many dermatologists and plastic surgeons have now launched their own skin-care lines (mine is Dr. Michelle Copeland Skin Care™), culled from the hundreds they've tried over the years. The formulations of these products tend to be halfway between OTC and prescription strength, and can be extremely effective. (For more information, visit www.drmichelle copelandskincare.com, or www.drcopeland.com.)

4. Sun Protection

In the summer I tend to cultivate a light suntan, and not a few of my patients have commented on it (one even says it keeps me "real"). I am an outdoors person: I enjoy gardening, swimming, biking, and jogging, and I walk a mile to work every day. Like most people, I love how the sun feels on my skin. So I suppose it *does* make me real in that I can empathize with my patients' bad sun habits. (It's the very rare person who, before stepping outside on a bright winter morning, remembers to cover his or her face with sunblock.) But I am smart about the amount of time I spend outdoors, and the kind of protection I wear. Sun penetrates cloud cover and even clothing, so you don't need much exposure at all to get even a little bit of color.

But tanning and burning are only the most immediately *visible* signs of sun damage. Permanent underlying damage, to both cells and their DNA, occurs every time the skin absorbs the sun's ultraviolet light. Some cells are killed immediately; others that are damaged spew chemicals that irritate tiny blood vessels, causing inflammation and redness. UV light also breaks down the skin's collagen and elastin fibers, which leads to sagging. And UV rays can alter cellular DNA and eventually cause skin cancer. So, long after the tan fades, genetic damage remains in the form of brown spots, uneven coloring, wrinkling, and pre-cancerous changes in cells.

Not a pretty picture. How do you deal with it?

The most effective way to stave off damage, short of avoiding the sun entirely, is to wear a broad-spectrum sunscreen any time you're outdoors. Developed fairly recently, a broad-spectrum formula blocks both ultraviolet-B light (the rays that burn) and the longer-wave ultraviolet-A light, which penetrates the skin more deeply. Not all sunscreens shield against both types of light. The most effective products contain zinc oxide—the white stuff that lifeguards wear on their noses, now available in a clear formula—which is considered a "physical barrier" because it's completely impervious to sunlight. It also acts as an antioxidant, helping to reduce the sun's harmful effects, and is extremely unlikely to elicit an allergic reaction. Titanium dioxide is another effective broad-spectrum physical barrier. Avobenzone, also known as Parsol 1789, is a fairly new chemical block that also screens out both UVA and UVB rays, but it breaks down over several hours, requiring frequent reapplication, and not uncommonly causes an allergic reaction.

There is a lot of confusion over how much SPF is enough. *SPF is a rating system that measures a sunscreen's effectiveness in protecting against sunburn-causing UVB rays only.* An SPF of 10 suggests you can stay in the sun ten times longer without burning than you could with no protection. However, we now know that sun damage will occur long before your skin even appears to burn. So I recommend wearing a minimum of 30 if you're outdoors much of the day, and 15 if you're outside infrequently—and replenishing it often.

Fortunately, there are now lots of daily face creams that contain SPFs (typically offering protection of 15) but that don't leave the skin feeling greasy or sticky. If you have sensitive skin, opt for a fragrance-free sunscreen labeled "hypoallergenic" or "non-stinging." A nonchemical sunblock—one that contains zinc oxide or titanium dioxide—is also safe for all skins.

Your skin is the clothing that nature gave you. If you've abused it (as most of us have, to one degree or another), then cleansing, exfoliating, moisturizing, and using sun protection provide ways to undo the damage. In the next chapter, we'll look at some of the latest skin-saving technologies that help to iron out the wrinkles and irregularities that inevitably occur over time.

6

The "Lunchtime" Solution: Getting Rid of Wrinkles

Sometimes I joke that I'm like a personal trainer. Many of my patients schedule me once or even twice a week for a little "tweak." One day they might come for a light-laser peel to smooth out fine facial lines; another day they'll want a fat injection to plump up their flattened cheeks. Some routinely book me a couple of weeks in advance of a wedding, vacation, or special event for which they want to look their best. My patients are busy people, and available hours are so few and precious that many won't give up even the short recovery times promised by mini-lifts, mini-tucks, and other small-incision surgeries. They want to look good *now*.

Thanks to continued advances in lasers, soft-tissue fillers, and other technologies, there are now a number of one-hour "lunchtime fixes" for worry lines, crow's-feet, and loose skin that can be done right in the office using no (or a mild local) anesthesia. After such a procedure, you can return to work the same afternoon. These procedures may be all you really need to feel better about how you look. They're so quick and minimally invasive, in fact, that I've done some of them, from start to finish, on TV shows on which I've been a guest. You're left with no scars, raw surfaces, or noticeable swelling. Will you see the full effect the same day? Not always, but you'll see it soon, and you'll have zero downtime, which makes these solutions so appealing.

Of course, you needn't have these lunchtime fixes done at lunchtime, but many of my most harried patients do come in on their break from work. In fact, it's the perfect time for undergoing certain procedures because, for instance, you can't nap after a Botox injection: Liquid Botox is injected into muscles, and if, immediately after, you lay your head on a pillow for a significant period, the substance can absorb unevenly.

Best of all, perhaps, is that these quick fixes don't cost the thousands of dollars that surgical procedures do. Laser treatments run $350 to $500 per session; Botox injections tend to cost $400 to $500 for an area; and soft-tissue fillers run from $350 to $900 a visit, depending on the type and number of sites treated.

A SURGERY-PHOBE GOES FOR THE QUICK FIX

After a summer of beachgoing and schlepping her kids to and from day camp, Lianne, a forty-two-year-old mother of two, began to notice signs of wear and tear on her skin. "I was starting to get a few lines around my mouth and eyes," she said, "but I didn't think I was ready for a face-lift. Besides, I'm terrified of surgery and would do anything to avoid it."

Still relatively young and in good health, Lianne had excellent skin quality, with little underlying sagging. I proposed smoothing out her finer wrinkles with microdermabrasion, treating her crow's-feet with the muscle-relaxant Botox, and using fat injections to fill in the deeper lines around her mouth and chin.

"The microdermabrasion made my pores tighter and caused my skin to reflect light in a more flattering way," recalls Lianne. "When I left the doctor's office, I had only a bit of puffiness around my mouth and stiffness near my eyes, but no pain whatsoever." Since receiving her first treatments more than a year ago, Lianne has been back for fat injections once and for Botox three times. "The effect is quite subtle, which is how I want it," she says. "After a few weeks, people started to pay me compliments. Recently, my husband and I were sitting at a candlelight dinner when he leaned over and whispered, 'My God, you look twenty-five.' What woman isn't going to keep it up if her husband says that? There's no magical cure for wrinkles, but this comes close."

As we age, our faces begin to show the effects of gravity, sun damage, and the habitual movements of squinting, frowning, and chewing. The underlying tissues that keep skin taut and youthful start to break down, and wrinkles begin to appear all over the face, especially in the form of crow's-feet, laugh and frown lines, and droopy nasolabial folds (the lines that run diagonally from the corners of the nose to the sides of the mouth). Except perhaps for the handsomely etched, weathered cowboy, we all want these flaws to disappear.

One of the great advances in skin resurfacing is that we have such a wide choice of techniques to deal with problems, and patients always prefer having a choice—to determine which technique may best suit their needs, based on their particular problem or skin type. Also, as the surgeon, I don't feel straitjacketed to pick just one technique per patient. Often, the most effective solution is a combination of various resurfacing treatments.

Patients maintain their skin this way for years. If you start young, it's even possible that you can avoid ever being a candidate for surgery—though these techniques address only the skin's surface and its inner layers, not the musculature and fasciae under the skin, which are responsible for drooping.

SKIN RESURFACING TECHNIQUES

Microdermabrasion: Smoothing the Skin

Until recently, one of the most common skin-smoothing and rejuvenating methods was a process called dermabrasion, in which deep wrinkles were buffed away by an abrasive, rotating brush (think of a furniture sander and you will get the idea). While effective on deep wrinkles, especially around the mouth and nose, dermabrasion carried a risk of scarring, and left the face raw and red for weeks.

In the last couple of years, a kinder, gentler form of the technique has evolved called microdermabrasion. Although it won't get rid of deeper grooves like its more aggressive cousin, it is very effective at minimizing fine lines, large pores, acne scars, and pigment irregularities. There's even growing evidence that it can help eliminate outbreaks of adult acne. Microdermabrasion is also ideal for use on the neck, where the skin is thinner and carries a higher risk of scarring than on the face. Since its inception, the technique has really taken off—over 800,000 procedures were performed in 2001, up 35 percent from the previous year.

Rather than a sander, a narrow instrument is employed in microdermabrasion, one that sprays fine crystals at the skin and then, with a tiny vacuum, sucks them up along with the skin particles. Your surgeon will vary the speeds, depending on the part of the face he or she is treating and the particular problem—a little lighter to improve pore appearance or fine wrinkles; deeper if the patient has, say, pre-cancerous skin-cell changes or more pronounced sun damage. Microdermabrasion doesn't hurt, though it doesn't tickle, either: One patient compared it to a salt scrub.

Best of all, because of the suction mechanism, skin does not scab or flake off after treatment. However, microdermabrasion does need to be repeated four to six times before results are evident. I've had astonishingly good outcomes with this method—some patients' skin becomes so tight and glowing that they look as if they could have had a face-lift! Microdermabrasion is even gentle enough for patients with darker skin.

One session of microdermabrasion costs $250 to $400.

"Light Touch" Lasers: Tightening the Skin

There are so many varieties of lasers for different functions that even an expert has trouble keeping them straight. There are lasers for skin resurfacing, for hair removal, for vein zapping, and for eliminating age spots. The laser functions vary depending on their wavelength, duration of pulse, and where the pulse is directed.

For some time we've used ablative lasers for smoothing deep wrinkles and heavily mottled or pockmarked skin. Ablative means "removing by vaporization or melting"; ablative lasers takes off the top layer of photodamaged skin, encouraging the growth of healthy new cells. There are two common types of ablative lasers. The older type, the **carbon dioxide (CO_2)** laser, functions by projecting CO_2 at skin cells and demolishing them. It leaves the face very raw and red for weeks (sometimes even months) and carries a significant risk of scarring. Developed more recently, the **Erbium** laser works when its energy is absorbed by the water in skin cells, causing shrinkage and a change in the underlying collagen. It is less injurious to the skin than the CO_2 laser, though it can also cause redness that lingers for quite some time.

What if you don't have several weeks to go into hiding and heal? Enter the new generation of **non-ablative or "light touch" lasers,** which only imperceptibly remove the top layer of skin. What they do—in an hour—is use a thermal effect to stimulate changes in the elastic tissue deep within the skin, resulting in generalized tightening.

Apart from temporary redness, these non-ablative lasers (including Nd:YAG, Alexandrite, and Pulsed Dye) carry a very small risk of side effects, and patients can return to work immediately after treatment. Over the course of several treatments there will be a reorganization of the collagen cells beneath the skin, resulting in a tighter, more youthful texture. This is an ideal solution for those with mild to moderate wrinkling and a little sagging. Patients prefer it to ablative lasers because it's less painful—some brands, like CoolTouch, emit a cooling spray to protect the skin, they heal more quickly after treatment, and they won't walk around for months looking like they just got the worst sunburn of their lives. Whereas ablative lasers aren't advised for use on ethnic skins because of the risk of permanent lightening and scarring, light touch lasers are safe for people of every skin color. A treatment costs from $350 to $500 per session.

Your doctor may recommend yet another wrinkle-reducing method, called **Intense Pulsed Light (IPL).** While technically not a laser, IPL uses multiple wavelengths of light to achieve its effects. It triggers collagen growth, and treats pigmentation issues such as rosacea and age spots in one fell swoop. Because it is "nonspecifically directed" (meaning its light is diverted to many targets at once), the results are much more subtle, and it may require multiple sessions to see significant change. The cost is comparable to that of laser treatment. There are a few techniques on the horizon that may compete with light-laser treatments, including radiofrequency energy, but for now, lasers are the best thing I know of to promote collagen growth and reduce wrinkling nonsurgically.

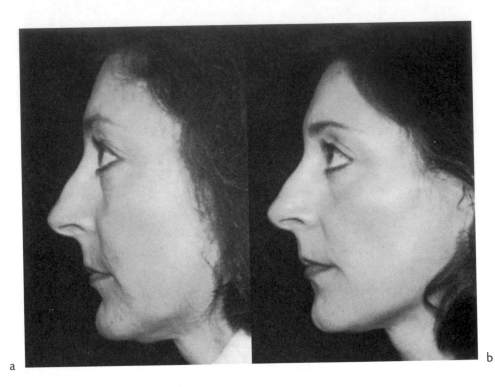

a

b

MICRODERMABRASION AND LIGHT-LASER TREATMENTS

This forty-nine-year-old lawyer came to me expecting to have plastic surgery to tighten the skin in her cheek and jowl area (a). Because the sagging wasn't dramatic and her skin quality was good, however, I suggested we start instead with microdermabrasion and light-laser treatments. Half a year later (b), you can really see the improvement.

The Combo Platter

For greatest effect, however, I like to use these two techniques in combination: microdermabrasion to smooth the skin's surface, and light touch laser to tighten the underlying connective tissues. In skin where aging is the main grievance (rather than, say, large pores or acne scars), it seems pointless to me to improve only the skin's texture, or only its sagginess, when microdermabrasion and laser treatment together can have such dramatic effects.

There are other combination treatments that make good skin sense. I might also follow microdermabrasion with a Botox injection to freeze more prominent crow's-feet or frown lines (you can read more about Botox later in this chapter). Or I might apply external ultrasound, a technique that shapes subcutaneous fat, to the neck area to help minimize jowls.

It is worth raising these "combo" options with your doctor and exploring how techniques can be used synergistically to achieve the result you want.

QUOTE, UNQUOTE

"I have a light, Irish complexion, and I had developed quite a bit of sun damage from living in the South for much of my life. I've also been a runner for 20 years, and probably haven't worn sunblock as religiously as I should have. My skin looked worn out, and was flecked with sun spots. I decided to get a series of microdermabrasion and light-laser treatments. I could see the difference right away once the skin healed: It was tighter and softer to the touch. Last spring, I was back in Ireland for some time. I have a friend over there, an artist, and at one point I caught him staring at my face. 'Did you get a face-lift?' he finally blurted out. He had trouble believing I hadn't."

—Audrey, 57, homemaker

THE INJECTABLE SOLUTION: SOFT-TISSUE FILLERS

Soft-tissue fillers—most commonly injectable bovine or human collagen and fat—can help fill in facial lines and creases, resulting in a temporarily more youthful appearance. When injected below the skin, these fillers plump up wrinkled or sunken areas of the face and add fullness to the cheeks and lips. Botox injection, the most popular procedure I perform, employs a toxin to paralyze underlying muscles and thus relaxes wrinkles. While the effects of these methods are temporary and require returning for refresher injections every few months, the results are so dramatic that many people actually enjoy these regular cosmetic tune-ups. "So long as I can put off a surgical procedure, I'm going to keep getting Botox for the next few years," says Lianne.

A word of caution: Because such procedures are so easy to perform, cosmetic surgeons aren't the only ones who perform them. Dermatologists, facialists, and spa technicians now do them, too. Before you receive treatment, verify that your practitioner is licensed to administer the procedure, and has the experience and referrals to prove it. I've heard too many stories of patients winding up in the hospital with a raging infection because of unsanitary conditions or the practitioner's incompetency.

Collagen

Collagen helps make skin strong. It's a protein that lends firmness to the connective tissue beneath the skin's surface. But sun exposure breaks down collagen, as does age. As we get older, we need outside help to keep our skin taut. If we could plump up the collagen from within the face and make wrinkles appear less deep, then we'd be in business. For that to happen, though, we might as well wait for the cows to come home, right?

Exactly. This is where the cattle come in.

Bovine collagen has long been considered the gold standard for filling light wrinkles. A fibrous substance, it is extracted from cowhide and "harvested" (purified), turned into liquid form, and mixed with a local anesthetic. This solution is then used as an injectable filler for humans—so long as they're not allergic to it.

How do you know if you are allergic? At least a month before your first treatment, a tiny sample of bovine collagen is injected into your forearm. If redness, swelling, or itching occur within three weeks, then you're not a candidate for this method. If, like most people, you show no reaction, then you're cleared to receive the treatment. The liquid collagen is injected into the areas to be plumped—typically, the fine lines around the mouth, the eyes, between the eyebrows, and in the lips. The solution contains lidocaine, a local anesthetic, so the injection isn't painful, though it may pinch. (Collagen injected into the lips, which are more sensitive, may hurt a bit more.) Start to finish, the procedure takes less than ten minutes per injection, and runs $350 to $750 for each site.

Afterward, there may be minor swelling. Cold compresses and hydrocortisone help to reduce inflammation and redness; makeup can be used to cover discoloration, which won't last longer than a few hours. Complications, which are very rare, include infection, scarring, and allergic reaction. Asymmetries are correctible with another office visit. *Caution: If you're pregnant or suffer from an autoimmune disease or a connective-tissue disease like rheumatoid arthritis or scleroderma, you should avoid collagen altogether.*

The biggest problem with collagen—and it's why I now use it less often than I do some other fillers—is that it doesn't last terribly long. For some people, the effect will last only a couple of months; for others, whose bodies don't absorb the collagen so quickly, results endure for up to nine months. I do have patients who are big fans, though, and who refuse to consider anything else.

URGENT QUESTION:
IS BOVINE COLLAGEN SAFE?

Although bovine collagen injections have never been linked to a human case of mad-cow disease (bovine spongiform encephalopathy), some patients express concern. To allay your fears, ask your doctor to make sure that the wrinkle filler is from a company with documented anti-contamination standards. Zyderm and Zyplast, the only current FDA-approved injectable collagens, are taken from closed herds of cows that have been raised on an isolated California ranch. No case of BSE has yet been found in U.S. cattle.

Autologous Fat Transfer

Autologous simply means "your own." And who doesn't have a little fat to spare? Using a cannula—a small probing tube attached to a tiny vacuum—the surgeon liposuctions out a little bit of fat, usually from the buttocks, hips, or abdomen; cleanses it with a saline solution; and injects the fat into the face. It may sound like a literal pain in the butt, but the procedure is quick and not particularly painful, since it is done under local anesthesia. Just this past week, Judith, a patient of mine, came in for a little plumping up a few days before attending her twenty-fifth college reunion. She wanted to make her lips fuller and to soften her laugh lines, and we used her own fat to do so. First I lipoed 100 cubic centimeters out of her hip, then I cleansed it and injected it right

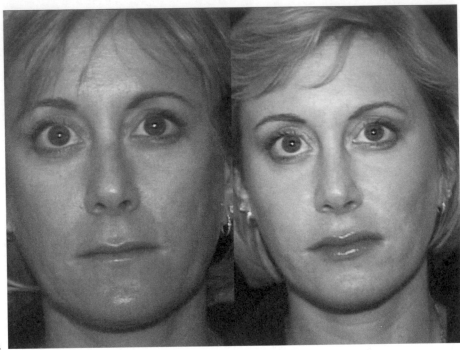

a   b

AUTOLOGOUS FAT INJECTIONS

Whenever this public relations representative lost weight, it came off her face, leaving her looking drawn and aged (a). At thirty-nine, she felt she was too young for surgery, so we liposuctioned her hips and injected the fat into her lips, cheeks, and nasolabial folds through the inside of her lip—a technique I developed. Just one week later, (b) her face is fuller and younger looking.

into her face. Judith walked into my office at eleven and walked out at noon, with only a little bit of swelling and a face that looked fabulous, refreshed, and ready to greet her former classmates.

Autologous fat makes the best filler for several reasons: It came out of you, so you can't be allergic to it; it offers greater versatility than bovine collagen and can be used in more areas of the face; and it lasts longer than the other fillers—about 50 percent of the fat stays permanently where it was injected. Then there's the added bonus of losing a smidgen of fat from the body part of your choice. Your doctor can even remove extra fat to freeze, for use up to six

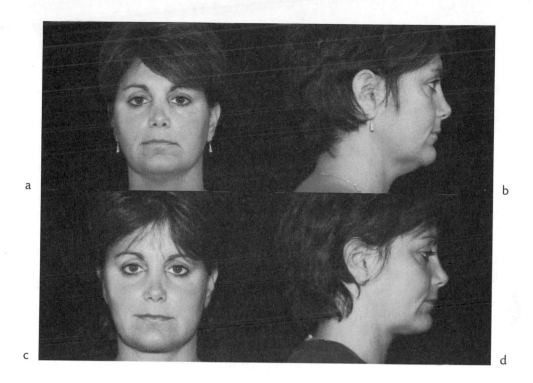

a   b
c   d

NECK LIPECTOMY AND FAT INJECTIONS

This thirty-eight-year-old ad sales manager wanted to do something about her thin lips and deep laugh lines (nasolabial folds), as well as her emerging wattle (a), (b). I tightened her neck with a neck lipectomy (see Chapter 8). Then, using fat injections, I plumped up her cheeks, nasolabial folds, and lips. As a result of her new filled-out face, even her eyes look brighter (c), (d).

---

months later. Fat does have limitations, though. While it's ideal for filling deeper grooves in the nasolabial folds and chin, and for plumping up lips and cheeks, it's not particularly effective on fine lines.

If the areas to be plumped are in or around the lips or chin, I inject fat on the *inside* of the lip. My patients love this approach, because it leaves no marks on the face. Otherwise, the injection is made into the areas that need fattening, leaving a tiny, temporary pinprick scab.

The whole job, including lipo, takes less than an hour. Your face will look somewhat swollen afterward—more so than after a collagen injection—

because we need to "overcorrect" and inject twice as much fat into a given area than is needed to fill it. Why? Because fat can be surprisingly elusive, and not all of the injected fat will stay in place. Indeed, within a week of the procedure, nearly half of the relocated fat will be reabsorbed by your body. If you don't overcorrect, you'll just be back in the office a week later requesting another injection.

Plan to spend between $1,000 and $3,000 for this procedure.

WARNING: STEALTH SILICONE

Not long ago, liquid silicone was the favorite injectable filler of some doctors. While a few still use it, liquid silicone has never received FDA approval for injection purposes, as it can cause local irritation and inflammation. Also—and more important—once silicone is injected, it is very difficult to remove from the tissue. If a problem should arise, correcting it is tough. I never use it and don't recommend it.

Human Collagen

One of the newest injectable fillers on the market, human collagen offers the best of both worlds. Because it's derived from human cadavers, you don't have to be tested for allergic reaction as with bovine collagen (it is about as disease-free as you can get, provided the company adheres to the American Tissue Bank Association Guidelines). Furthermore, you get a smoother line with human collagen, and it seems to last longer—six months to a year.

I use human collagen a lot (one popular brand name you may encounter is Fascian, which also contains processed connective tissue). It's particularly effective in treating nasolabial folds, lines above the lips, frown lines, smile lines, and even acne pitting, and carries a standard risk of infection or scarring if not administered correctly.

Directly after treatment, you may find that your skin is slightly red or bruised at the injection site, and a bit lumpy. Individual treatments cost from $500 to $900.

Goretex

Yes, it's the same material that windbreakers are made of. Goretex is a filler, though, and not injected. It's actually *threaded* into the lips through a small incision at the corner of the mouth. I don't favor its use, because the lips are (or should be) soft and supple, and it seems counterproductive to put something firm in them. While Goretex will give the desired appearance of plumpness, it's not pleasant to touch or kiss. Plus, there have been reports of scar tissue formation.

Hyaluronic Acid and Other Fillers for the Future

New wrinkle-reducing fillers are always emerging. One getting a lot of buzz is Hyaluronic acid, from the connective tissue derived from plants or grown in a lab (brands include Restylane and Perlane). Hyaluronic acid has been used successfully for years in Europe and is awaiting FDA approval. So is Artecoll, synthetic beads of Plexiglas mixed with collagen, which is supposed to offer permanent plumping. Scientists are even developing tissue-engineering techniques, where fat cells are cultivated as stem cells and cultivated for various uses, including injectable fillers. There are sure to be many other treatments on the market before long. Be sure that the filler you choose is FDA-approved for the purpose for which your doctor is using it, and that he or she is licensed to do so. In just two years' time, we'll undoubtedly have many more options that deliver even more satisfying and long-lasting results.

BOTOX: THE MOST POPULAR PROCEDURE I DO

Technically, Botox isn't a filler at all but a chemical that weakens or paralyzes the facial muscles used for movement (such as those between or at the sides of your eyes). As fillers and quick fixes go, Botox (or botulinum toxin, a product of bacteria) is one of the best things around. It can have a profound effect on the face, especially on fine wrinkles. It can eliminate a young mother's perpetually angry scowl, or a reformed sun-worshipper's crow's-feet. Botox was approved by the FDA for cosmetic use only last year, but even before that, it had surged in popularity: During 2001, more than 1.2 million Botox procedures were performed, a phenomenal 2,204-percent jump since 1997. I'm such a proponent of Botox that I inject it into myself—in my crow's-feet, my forehead, and the furrows between my eyes.

Rather than "plumping" like collagen and fat, Botox blocks the impulses that nerves send to muscles, essentially paralyzing the muscles and diminishing their ability to tense. Because of this, it is especially effective in improving the vertical "scowl lines" many people get between the eyebrows. Because these furrows tend to be deep, I sometimes recommend using a combination of Botox and a filler, such as fat or collagen. Botox can also be effective on the nasolabial folds (the lines radiating from nose to mouth)—but be warned that in rare cases, the injection may hamper a patient's ability to smile or even speak by causing temporary paralysis of the mouth muscles. Recently, we have started using Botox also on the lines around the neck's platysma muscles (those prominent vertical bands) with great results.

Using a very fine needle, the surgeon injects Botox in small doses where the facial muscles are most active—between the eyebrows and at the sides of the eyes, or beside the mouth. After receiving treatment, you're forbidden to lie down for several hours, because the medicine can absorb unevenly. You may have a headache or some local tingling or bruising at the injection site, though this is rare. It takes one to three days to see the effects, and the treated area will continue to improve for up to two weeks. That's when I schedule my patients to return, to see if a touch-up is needed.

Complications are rare with Botox, though it can drift beyond the target area so that, for example, one eyelid droops until the treatment wears off. Because Botox was the first bacterial toxin to be used as a medicine, it underwent one of the strictest approval trials ever conducted by the FDA and is very safe.

Botox tends to be effective for four to six months, so if you like the effect, you'll need to come back for regular visits. There have been reports of people building up tolerance to Botox, but that's also unusual. In the future, we will surely see the introduction of other new wrinkle-erasing substances; even now, trials are under way of a new Botox derivative called Myobloc.

One more word of caution: Because of Botox's incredible surge in popularity, a lot of folks want it—and a lot of people are willing to inject you with it. One growing (and slightly disturbing) trend is Botox parties, where guests eat, drink, and get a needle between the eyes. Lack of regulation has become a problem. But medicine is not a parlor game: If you're not having Botox injected by a licensed practitioner, such as a plastic surgeon or dermatologist, then make sure the procedure is being done in a sterile fashion, and that the Botox being used has been kept in a freezer and is freshly mixed for your treatment.

Plan to spend $400 to $500 to treat one area.

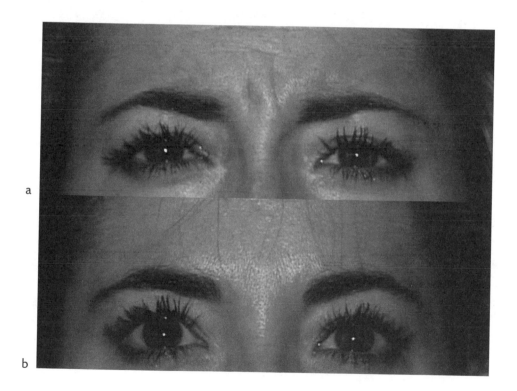

a

b

BOTOX INJECTIONS

People told this thirty-year-old public relations professional that she looked angry all the time (a). Botox injections took care of the furrows between her eyebrows. One month after her treatment, there is little trace of those forehead worry lines (b).

THE BONUS BENEFITS OF BOTOX

As Botox's popularity increased, it was found to have unexpected uses: It can eliminate migraines when injected in the forehead. In fact I have patients, including my nurse, who get the treatment for that reason alone. Other reports suggest that Botox, when injected in the armpits and hands, may prevent excessive sweating, because muscles associated with the sweat glands are relaxed by the substance. Who knows what other benefits we'll discover next?

HOW DO I KNOW WHICH
WRINKLE TREATMENT IS RIGHT FOR ME?

Are you a candidate for Botox, fat, or collagen? It depends on the depth of your wrinkles, on your budget, and on your willingness to come back for refills. Here's a breakdown:

Source	Best for . . .	Pros	Cons
Collagen (Cow hooves)	. . . filling in fine wrinkles around the eyes, nose, and mouth	Widely available; less expensive than other fillers	Potential allergic reaction in 3 to 10 percent of patients; results last only 3 to 9 months
Human Collagen (Human cadavers)	. . . filling in fine lines around the nose, lips, and eyes, and acne scars	Smooth appearance; no allergy risk; lasts longer than collagen	Injected with a larger needle
Autologous fat (Buttocks, abdomen, or hips)	. . . plumping up deeper grooves around nasolabial folds, cheeks, and lips	Safest of the fillers; mostly permanent	Requires liposuction to "harvest" fat, increasing procedure time; need for "overcorrection" means face is swollen for days
Goretex (Synthetic)	. . . plumping up the lips by threading	None, as far as I'm concerned	A stiff lip that looks and feels unnatural

Source	Best for . . .	Pros	Cons
Botox (Botulinum toxin A)	. . . relaxing crows'-feet, nasolabial folds, forehead frown lines, and neck bands	Quick, relatively affordable; no downtime	Requires replenishing every 4–6 months; risk of droopy eyelid or inability to smile if toxin leaks
Hyaluronic acid (Connective tissue from plants, bacteria)	Filling in fine wrinkles around eyes, lips, and nose	No allergic risk, gives smooth appearance	Ideally needs to be repeated; as of this printing, not yet FDA approved

As you can see, there is much that can be done in a short amount of time to diminish wrinkles, lines, grooves, and other signs of aging that make you look tired, angry, and therefore older than necessary. The next chapter discusses a few more "lunchtime" solutions that can eliminate ugly blemishes and boost your self-image along with your appearance.

7 | Other Quick Fixes: Blemish Busters

Ironing out wrinkles using lasers, fillers, and resurfacing techniques are just some of the ways we can help improve your appearance quickly, predictably, and at a relatively low cost. Ugly age spots, annoying spider veins, and persistent hair growth can also be eliminated with a flick of a laser. Got a lunch hour or two, or three? The fix is in.

SUN AND AGE SPOTS

How do sun spots, age spots, and liver spots form? (They're all the same thing, by the way.) By exposure to the sun. Melanin, a pigment, is produced by skin cells. Sun stimulates its production; the more that's produced, the more pigment that becomes visible in our skin. And as we get older, our tendency to form pigment increases.

Sun and age spots form not only on the face, but are particularly pesky on the hands and chest—areas we often forget to cover with sunblock. Lots of patients come to me for treatment of their hands, in particular, because even if your face looks youthful, a mottled, liver-spotted hand can add years to your appearance.

To improve or eliminate these spots, your doctor may start with exfoliation techniques such as acid peels and microdermabrasion (described in the previous two chapters) to encourage the skin's cells to turn over. However, individual spots can be targeted as well using quick, painless techniques:

◆ **Pigment Blockers.** These work by inhibiting the skin's production of melanin. The most popular creams contain the ingredient hydroquinone or kojic acid. Certain natural herbs, like thyme, also help to block pigment, though less effectively. It will take roughly four to six weeks to see the full effect of these blockers, but, as with exfoliation, pigment production eventually will even out.

◆ **Lasers.** Spot-removal lasers (including Pulsed Dye and Q-Switched) work by vaporizing the pigment in skin. Patients report little discomfort during this procedure, although a topical anesthetic can be used. The treatment causes flaking and the spots scab over, but underneath the pigment vanishes. How bad are the scabs? It depends on their location on the body. One patient had to take a business trip to Europe with five or six scabs on her hands; she felt perfectly comfortable just telling her colleagues she'd had some sun spots removed. Another patient with a very fair, Irish complexion had several age spots removed from her face. She recalls, "My Aunt Marie was sitting outside in the waiting room—it was her turn next. I walked out and she gasped. 'I'll put it to you this way,' she told me, 'if you sat down next to me on the bus, I'd get off right away!'" Fortunately, these small scabs fall off within a week or so.

You will likely need more than one treatment to get rid of a particularly stubborn spot. Spot laser treatments cost $350 to $500 per session.

YOUR SKIN DURING PREGNANCY

Pregnancy can wreak havoc on the skin. Hormonal changes and weight gain can cause hyperpigmentation, stretch marks, and accelerated skin growth. For the most part, women are genetically predisposed to certain conditions, but there are things we can do to help skin regain its youthful, pre-pregnancy look. For instance:

- **Stretch marks.** I tell my pregnant patients to moisturize their growing bellies so the skin's collagen and elastin layers stay healthy and resist thinning. The more rapid the weight gain, of course, the greater the likelihood of stretch marks. Post-pregnancy acid creams encourage exfoliation of dead skin, and help the skin to regain its glow. I sometimes use microdermabrasion on stretch marks, but it requires multiple treatments over a large area—and lots of patience. Some light lasers can also help tighten stretch marks. When sagging and scarring are really bad, though, I usually advocate a tummy tuck.

- **Pregnancy "mask."** The cocktail of hormones coursing through a pregnant woman's body can boost pigment production, especially when the skin is exposed to sun. Some women even get wide brown patches on their face, known as the "mask of pregnancy." This is most easily eliminated post-pregnancy through repeated acid peels and/or laser treatments.

- **Skin tags.** Again, hormones rev up skin cell production, which may result in the growth of tiny flaps of skin, especially around the face, neck, and chest. Your surgeon can easily excise these manually.

SPIDER VEINS

At least half of all women get spider veins (known as *telangiectasias* or *sunburst varicosities*), those ugly mini-roadmaps of wine-red and blue lines just beneath the surface of the skin, generally found in the face (particularly around the nose and cheeks), thighs, and lower leg. Fortunately, we can easily zap them away with lasers.

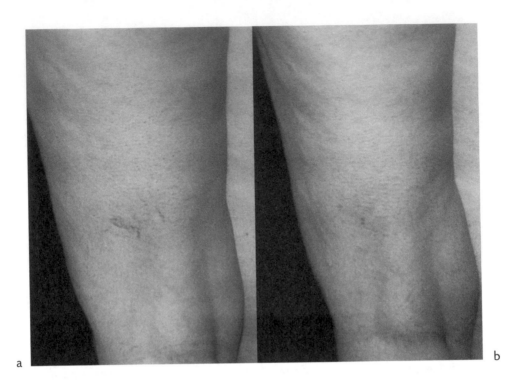

a   b

SPIDER VEIN REMOVAL

Bothered by broken blood vessels on her legs (a), this forty-eight-year-old lawyer was embarrassed to wear shorts or a bathing suit in the summer. After just two treatments with the VersaPulse laser (b), you can really see a difference!

The cause of spider veins is largely genetic, though other culprits include pregnancy, standing or sitting for long stretches, fluctuations in weight, and the use of birth-control pills. The veins and broken capillaries, though ugly, are superficial. They connect to other, larger veins—but frankly, you don't need them to function.

In the old days a needle was used to coagulate the blood vessel, which eliminated it, but this also caused minor scarring. The next solution was to inject a saline medication (with other chemicals) into the veins to irritate them and ultimately to cause the blood vessels to collapse. Unfortunately, the chemicals could leak, causing irritation and discoloration. Finally, laser technology was developed that allows us to eliminate spider veins without irritation or downtime.

Vein-zapping is a simple, painless procedure. The doctor aims the laser at the offending vein cluster. The laser has been programmed to target certain colors—in this case, purplish red. Once zapped, blood flow to the web of veins is cut off without affecting the surrounding skin. Without a blood source, the veins will collapse and disappear. The newest lasers allow us to work on larger blood vessels than we could before, and I'm confident that our ability to use lasers to deal with more problematic blood vessels, currently fixable only by surgery, is not far off. (Doctors may also treat spider veins with Intense Pulsed Light (IPL) which, though not technically a laser, uses multiple wavelengths of light to gently remove discoloration.)

The whole procedure takes about fifteen minutes. Afterward, each of the affected areas will be blemished purple, but the discoloration fades in several days. Topical cortisone cream and ice can help diminish mild swelling. Also, in a minority of cases, the lasered areas may appear brownish; this fades too, though it may take weeks to do so. (Pigment blockers can help reduce the splotchiness.) Avoid the sun both right before and right after treatment, or you risk developing color irregularities. Note that you may have to return for a second laser session to eliminate each cluster in its entirety.

A spider vein treatment costs $400 to $700 per session.

URGENT QUESTION:
WHAT CAN I DO ABOUT MY VARICOSE VEINS?

Until recently, the cure for varicose veins was almost as grisly as the condition itself. Removing those big hammocks of veins from the knees, thighs, and calves required surgery (known as "stripping") under general anesthesia, and an overnight hospital stay. Now the FDA has approved a procedure called Endoluminal Radio Frequency Elimination (ERFE). It involves inserting a wirelike catheter containing electrodes into the vein, which heats it, causing the vein to collapse. Because only local anesthesia is used, a patient can go right back to work. The fee is somewhere between $2,000 and $3,000, and may be covered by insurance if the veins are very painful or otherwise physically debilitating. Scientists are also developing a new generation of intravascular lasers to treat leg vessels of all sizes without requiring surgery.

HAIR REMOVAL

"Unwanted hair" has to be one of the more unpleasant two-word phrases in the English language. Fortunately, technological advances in the last few years are helping us to deal with the problem.

First, forget electrolysis. It's a highly imperfect remedy that works on one offending hair at a time and comes with a high risk of irritation from ingrowth and scarring. Lasers, especially the new breed, are far superior in removing hair via a process called **photo-epilation** (sometimes referred to by the laser types Diode, Long Pulse, Ruby, and nd:YAG). Laser hair removal has simplified the lives of thousands of people. We can do away with unsightly facial hair, leg hair, underarm hair, bikini-area growth, and for men, back and chest hair, in only a couple of treatments. Imagine going months without shaving or waxing!

How do hair-removal lasers work? Until very recently, one favored technique involved dying the hair follicles with a dark gel and vaporizing the pigment with a laser, disabling its growth potential. Unfortunately, the process couldn't guarantee total hair removal; it tended to be a little painful; and more than one treatment was needed to deactivate the hair over a large area.

A new generation of stronger lasers can now effect near-permanent hair removal after several treatments. For these lasers the skin isn't painted with gel; rather, laser light is directed at the melanin in the hair itself. This method is effective all over the body—arms, underarms, backs, legs, bikini line, mustaches, and other facial hair. Because these lasers have a "cool tip" and chill the skin around the area where they work their magic, they aren't particularly painful. There may be some ensuing skin irritation, however, which takes a week or so to go away. (If you're having your bikini line treated, don't schedule your appointment for the day before you plan to be at the pool.) Risks associated with the more intense lasers are few, but possible complications include reddening, local irritation, scabbing, and temporary skin discoloration.

Use of either type of laser takes fifteen minutes to one hour, depending on how large an area is being treated. Photo-epilation costs between $300 and $1,800, depending on the site.

SCAR REVISION

Whether a scar results from an accident or a previous surgery, for many people it is not a badge of courage but an unsightly or even deforming mark. In 5 to 10 percent of people, scars become hypertrophied because of an overproduction of scar tissue, and in some cases a keloid develops, causing a scar to appear dark, thickened, and raised. It used to be that to get rid of a scar, doctors had to excise it surgically and resuture the wound in such a way as to minimize its appearance. But that really meant just replacing one blemish with another one potentially just as noticeable.

Fortunately, today we have several ways to improve a scar's appearance. Some techniques are most effective when a scar is still fresh, such as pigment-blocking creams to even out color, silicone gel to improve texture, and massage to break down the tissue. But we also have several options after a scar has fully formed. Steroids injected directly into the healed wound can help to shrink the tissue, as can CO_2 lasers. Microdermabrasion can flatten the scar, while lasers can decrease the blood-vessel formation in the area and normalize color.

Laser and microdermabrasion treatments to smooth or improve the appearance of scars can cost anywhere from $150 to $500 per treatment.

TATTOO YOU: PERMANENT MAKEUP

Some of us can't go anywhere without freshening up a little—a touch of eye-liner, say, or a dash of lipstick. Wouldn't it be convenient to speed up your daily makeup routine, yet still look as you do after taking all that time and care? Imagine not having to worry about your makeup smudging or fading after eating a meal, or sweating from a workout, or being in the sun? If you can't see well enough to apply eyeliner, wouldn't it be nice to have it applied permanently?

Amazingly, eyeliner, eyebrow liner, eye shadow, lip liner, or lipstick can now be "tattooed" on the face, quickly and permanently. A tattoo not only gives you bolder color but also some structural definition that you've lost, or possibly never had. "I have little beady eyes, and now when I get up in the morning I don't look 'blank,'" says Lynne, who received permanent eyeliner. "The eyeliner opens my eyes, makes them appear larger, and thickens my lashes at the base. The treatment has cut down on my makeup time tremen-dously. If someone calls to say they're coming over, I can be ready right away."

How is the job done? There's fundamentally no procedural difference between the butterfly-on-the-shoulder one gets in a tattoo parlor and the per-manent eye makeup one gets from a cosmetic surgeon. Through a very small needle, pigment is injected into the lowest level of skin, right where you want the improvement—the eyebrow (near the hair follicles), the outline of the lips, or wherever. With your surgeon, you will choose both the pigment color and, where applicable, the thickness of the line. I generally recommend my patients be conservative and choose a light color and thin line, since they can always enhance them with a pencil.

This simple procedure takes an hour, and because it is administered with a topical or local anesthetic, the needle will likely not hurt. Afterward, it's important to keep the treated area scrupulously clean to minimize the risk of infection. Treatment costs can vary widely, but you can expect to spend some-thing in the neighborhood of $750 to $2,000 for lips, eyelids, or eyebrows.

Without casting aspersions on a tattooist's art, one caution: No licensing is needed to inject permanent makeup. Tattoo facilities are often unsterile, and if the practitioner doesn't know what he or she is doing, it's easy to botch a procedure, particularly around the eyes. I once had a patient who came to me for remedial help: The dye from her permanent eyeliner had leaked all over her face! If you're not going to a cosmetic surgeon, make sure you've done your research on the practitioner, checked whether the clinic is accredited, and talked, if possible, to satisfied clients.

URGENT QUESTION:
HOW CAN I REMOVE A TATTOO?

It used to be that if someone wanted to remove a skin tattoo, a surgeon excised it with a scalpel, usually in increments to help the tissue around it expand and cover the wound. Today, we can use laser removal. The laser light picks up the pigment and vaporizes it. It takes a series of treatments, and if a tattoo is very deep, there may be some scarring. But the method is far superior to that used in the old days, when we had to remove it surgically.

This is cosmetic wellness in the fast-paced twenty-first century. For you "tiptoers" out there, you've gone about as far as you can to eliminate wrinkles and blemishes without resorting to surgery. For those of you who are still skittish about going under the knife, there's no reason why you can't continue using quick fixes such as lasers, microdermabrasion, and injectable fillers to keep rejuvenating your look over and over again.

However, I think it's time to clear up some misconceptions about cosmetic surgery. As technology improves, procedures are becoming less and less disruptive to a busy person's life, and results are dramatically more natural. In the next section, I'll introduce the various popular surgical procedures we do today and show you which, if any, is right for you.

PART THREE

Surgical Solutions

8

The Face:
Make It Beautiful

A year ago, Lynne, a fifty-eight-year-old former legal assistant, came to see me about her face, which she felt was aging more rapidly than she was. "In the previous few years I had begun to sag here, there, and everywhere," Lynne complained. "My neck dropped pretty much from my chin down to my collarbone. If I tried to cover it up by wearing a turtleneck or scarf, it only made things worse by bunching up the skin. I was also starting to get crow's-feet around my eyes and small wrinkles on my forehead."

She had consulted a plastic surgeon near her home in Dallas, and he'd recommended a face-lift. Nonetheless, Lynne was reluctant:

"When the plastic surgeon told me I needed a face-lift, I wanted to get a second opinion. I remembered the suffering a friend endured after hers—I saw her a week later, and she was in so much pain. That scared me. What's more, I knew I wouldn't have time for such a protracted recovery, and my daughter, who works with celebrities and sees bad face-lifts all the time, was bitterly opposed to the operation. Still, I knew I needed to do something about my appearance—something a little less radical."

Just looking at Lynne's despairing but still youthful countenance, it was clear to me she didn't need a full face-lift. She still had good skin resiliency, and her problems didn't justify such a drastic measure. Instead, we agreed that I would do a neck liposuction and eyelid lift. The neck lipo would eliminate the jowly look that was bothering her, and the eye lift would brighten her smallish eyes while subtly eliminating some of the wrinkling that had started in that area. The surgery took an hour and a half. The tiny incisions under her chin and in the creases of her eyelids, once healed, were scarcely visible; the recovery was quick and the results were outstanding. Says Lynne:

"It amazed me that without removing any skin or leaving scars, my appearance could change so much. My neck had such nice definition and I could finally see my eyes again. My friends, and even my daughter, who was so dead set against my having surgery, say I look great. One friend who noticed a difference finally asked if I'd had a face-lift. I was so elated to be able to say no!"

KEEPING THE SECRET: IT'S NOT ABOUT YOUNGER; IT'S ABOUT *BETTER*

Like Lynne, many of my patients looking to rejuvenate their face are surprised to discover that a face-lift (clinical name: *rhytidectomy*) is just one option. They are also relieved: The face-lifts performed even ten years ago—the ones on some celebrities and public figures that make us cringe—were excessive, trying to undo, say, thirty years of aging in one operation. No one wants to appear "done," with the skin pulled back too severely and the eyebrows shaped like McDonald's arches. And most of my patients aren't even looking to turn back the clock more than a handful of years. As one of my patients in her seventies put it, "I don't want to look younger; I want to look *better*."

The traditional face-lift is still the bread and butter of most plastic surgeons; some doctors devote almost their entire practice to doing them. Many excellent surgeons swear by the time-tested results of the classic face-lift, and techniques have progressed to the point that the typical outcome is increasingly natural.

It's my philosophy, however, that less is more. A traditional face-lift still leaves a patient with two prominent scars in front of the ears and requires a

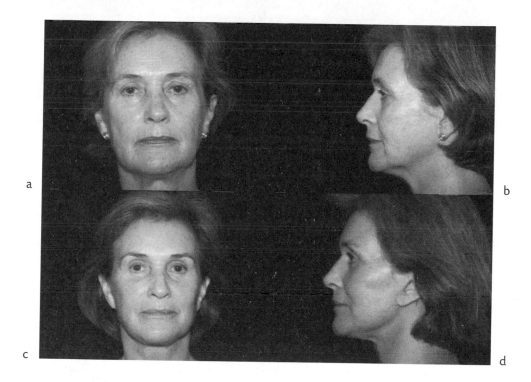

a

b

c

d

THE "OTHER" FACE-LIFT: A MINI-LIFT WITH ENDOSCOPIC FOREHEAD LIFT

I almost never do a traditional face-lift anymore—the results I get from a mini-lift combined with an endoscopic forehead lift are so fabulous, and the recovery so much easier, I don't see the point of doing more extensive surgery.

This sixty-four-year-old volunteer worker had sagging around the jowls, neck, and eyebrows (a,b), but was tentative about surgery because she was concerned about looking "done." As you can see, the effect is subtle, but dramatic: The brow lift raised her eyes (c), and the mini-lift tightened her lower face and highlighted her cheek area (d). I also injected her cheeks and lips with fat to plump them up. Wouldn't you agree that she looks terrific?

long recovery. Meanwhile, thanks to the advent of new technologies such as endoscopy (where surgery is done under the skin through a small incision using a tiny camera), liposuction, facial implants, and other "mini" procedures used either by themselves or in combination, we can do a lot less and achieve more positive, natural-looking results.

In fact, 95 percent of the face surgery I do is a suite of small procedures, and the final outcome is generally even better than what my patients used to enjoy with a full face-lift. Plus, because recovery is quicker, you won't feel conspicuous or worry that people will "find you out." I believe that facial surgery should be appreciated in the way one might appreciate the director of a good movie: While you watch the film, you're not aware of the director's presence, yet his or her contribution is evident in every frame. Similarly, after surgery, people shouldn't zero in on the feature that got "fixed" but rather sense the more rejuvenated, happier you, as expressed in your overall face.

ACKNOWLEDGING THAT YOU WANT FACIAL SURGERY

One of the biggest obstacles potential face-lift patients encounter is rationalizing why they're even considering having work done. *Why am I changing the face God gave me?* you may ask yourself. (And if *you* don't, someone close to you may volunteer the question.) Other doubts I hear all the time: *How can I justify rejecting the look of my family? Of my ethnic group?* And the ever-popular, *Just how vain* am *I?* I find these objections amusing; after all, is a shameless clotheshorse made to feel a fraction of the am-I-too-vain jolt that a face-lift candidate feels? Do we similarly stigmatize a woman who works out every single morning, without fail, or do we admire her? How about one who follows a strict skincare regimen morning, noon, and night? Or a woman who fixes her crooked teeth or dyes her prematurely gray hair?

Get over your guilt trip. Your face is you. It's your visual calling card; it inspires in others both first and last impressions. When you age and no longer feel as if your face accurately expresses who you are—when you look sad or angry or overworked or underslept—you're in danger of actually coming to assume those feelings. Lynne, the patient who opted to go with two smaller procedures in lieu of a face-lift, explains:

> "We communicate without words all the time. All those sags and bags do a number on you, and you start to feel and act as tired and draggy as you look. Others pick up on it, and intuitively know they can push you around. What I learned after my surgery is that if you look *more* vibrant, you tend to act *more*

confident. As a result, people actually listen to you and treat you with greater respect."

In short, a facial flaw can have major psychological repercussions. Even if no one else sees what you see—if there's no obvious physical "problem"—remember that you're having this surgery for *you*, or should be. We all age, if at different rates. And we all have different thresholds for tolerating the changes that come with time: the jowls, the wattle, the bags, the bumps, the wrinkles. You have to decide what you can live with—or want to live without.

FACE TIME

When should you have facial surgery? When you're unhappy with the way you look.

Do you slather on more makeup than you used to? Have you become a year-round hat-and-scarf wearer? Do you opt for glasses to camouflage the bags under your eyes instead of wearing contacts? Do you stand in front of the mirror and tug at your skin to see how you would look if you had work done?

So long as you understand and accept the risks and expense involved, there's no reason to slog through life with a face that makes you miserable. One fifty-three-year-old public relations executive claims it was a Christmas family photograph that triggered her Light-Bulb Moment and brought her into my office. "I love my father dearly and miss him terribly," says Patricia, who had a mini-lift and eyelid surgery, "but standing next to him in the photo it was so obvious that I'd inherited his jawline. Those jowls made me look less like his daughter and more like his wife! When I looked in the mirror, some-how I felt fine. But pictures don't lie." A mini-lift tightened Patricia's neck, and she no longer dreads family photo ops.

There's one more important argument in favor of facial surgery that I pose to patients on the fence: *If you start early, and small, you may avoid ever needing a big procedure later.*

One patient in her late twenties had a weak chin and thick neck that made her look overweight. After our consultation, I decided to perform a chin implant and neck lipectomy (where excess fat in the neck is removed, and the muscle is tightened). The only scar she had after her recovery was a tiny dot under her chin. I believe that because she had these procedures done when she was young, her neck and jawline may never droop to the point where she feels she needs further surgical intervention. If she'd waited for years to deal with the problem, however, it's possible that her entire lower face would have become severely lax, necessitating a full face-lift.

HOW THE FACE AGES

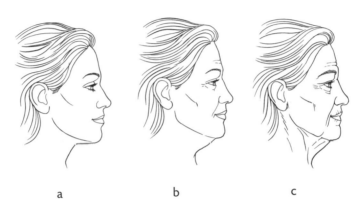

a   b   c

Skin resiliency diminishes with age. Sorry; we surgeons may be able to undo gravity's effects, but we can't stop it altogether. In adolescence, skin is plump and glowing. In our twenties (a), some aging and slight wrinkling (mostly from sun damage) has occurred, fine lines (such as frown lines) begin to appear, collagen and elasticity start to break down, and slight puffiness is evident around the eyes. In our thirties and forties (b), all of those changes become more pronounced and a "squaring off" of the face occurs. In our fifties and beyond (c), we experience a hollowing or increased puffiness in the eye area, laxity of the upper eyelid, the onset of jowls, and deeper, more pronounced nasolabial folds. Thanks to our common foe, gravity, a downward drift of the face continues unabated over the years.

Once upon a time, a person's age and corresponding skin resiliency determined the kinds of facial surgery he or she would get. But today, procedures once reserved for younger skin, such as liposuction and endoscopy, have proven effective on patients of all ages.

There are more than ten types of procedures I am likely to perform on those seeking facial rejuvenation. How do you know which you might need? Get a mirror and really give your face the third-degree, from crown to chin. Pinch, poke, and pull a little, then consult the chart below:

WHICH SURGERY IS RIGHT FOR YOU?

If you have ...	Then you may be a candidate for ...
Sagging cheeks Pronounced nasolabial folds (creases that run diagonally from the nose to the mouth) Jowls/softening in jaw area	Face-lift or mini-lift
Turkey-wattle neck Double chin	Neck lift or neck lipectomy
Sagging brows Horizontal forehead wrinkles Frown lines between the eyes	Forehead lift or endoscopic forehead lift
Baggy or droopy eyelids Puffy or fatty eyelids Lax lower eyelids	Eyelid lift
Weak chin Flat cheeks with minimal wrinkling	Facial implants

These procedures can be performed either by themselves or in combination, and are all fairly routine. My philosophy, as I've said, is to do as little as possible for the greatest possible benefit: You can always go back for more.

Now let's consider what to expect from the various face-enhancing procedures, including preparation, surgery, recovery, and possible post-operative side effects and complications.

TRADITIONAL FACE-LIFT (*RHYTIDECTOMY*)

While I almost never perform the traditional full face-lift anymore, there are plenty of doctors who do so regularly, and swear by them. Some may not be aware of the new small-incision and endoscopic techniques that have been pioneered and put into practice over the last five years; others may find they get perfectly satisfactory results with the method they've always used.

That said, there are several different types of face-lifts that doctors perform. A "skin-only" face-lift, which involves the removal and tightening of the skin without affecting the underlying tissues, yields only superficial—and usually temporary—results. A two-layer face-lift, the most common type, goes one step further, involving the tightening of the tissue under the skin, or SMAS (subcutaneous musculo-aponeurotic substance). A "deep-plane" face-lift reaches all the way down to the muscle near the bone. This kind of lift causes profound changes in appearance—too profound, for some—and carries a higher risk of nerve damage. Make sure you understand and discuss these differences with your surgeon before working with her or him to decide on an approach.

GETTING READY FOR FACE SURGERY

As with any procedure, you should avoid spicy or salty foods and alcohol (which promote inflammation) the day before surgery; steer clear of aspirin or other blood-thinning and anticoagulatory medications and anti-inflammatories, such as Advil or Motrin, for *two weeks prior*. (Make sure you go over your entire battery of medications with your surgeon before any procedure.) Read your doctor's pre-op instructions carefully, and consult Chapter 12 for more details. A couple of specific tips:

◆ If you dye your hair regularly, then you should have it done right before surgery; you won't be able to get a touch-up for at least a month afterward.

- Plan a comfortable wardrobe. You'll want clothing that can be put on easily after the procedure. Especially *verboten*: turtlenecks or sweaters that you have to pull over your head! I've received frantic calls from patients who've torn open their stitches while trying to work a tight neck over their ears just days after surgery.

- Prepare a convenient setup in your recovery room at home. You'll have to sleep with your head elevated for the first couple of days, so you'll need plenty of pillows. Some patients find sitting, and even sleeping, in an easy chair to be the most comfortable option.

What the Surgery Involves

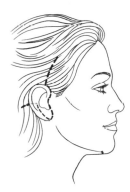

TRADITIONAL FACE-LIFT (RHYTIDECTOMY)

Face-lifts are now routinely performed in surgeons' offices on an outpatient basis, rather than in hospitals. Working on one side of the face at a time, the surgeon starts an incision inside the hairline at the temple, brings it down in front of the ear (some doctors take it behind the tragus, the little knob of flesh above the earlobe), and beneath the earlobe, continuing behind the ear and back into the hairline (see illustration). The scar may extend several inches into the hairline. During the procedure, the skin is separated from its underlying tissue, fat is removed, and the lax muscles and tissues of the face are pulled. The traditional lift tightens the face from the eyebrows all the way down to the chin at once. Surgery can take three to four hours, depending on its extent.

Many surgeons simultaneously tighten the neck when performing a face-lift (this is also true of the mini-lift). Technically, this is a neck lift (for more information on this procedure, see page 125). An incision is made under the chin, fat is removed, and the platysma muscles—the ones that stand out when you stretch your neck—are tightened.

There are distinct advantages to having a neck lift along with your face-lift: The incision is tiny and leaves virtually no scar; moreover, your smooth neck won't be out of sync with your youthful face (there's no bigger giveaway of a face-lift than a wrinkly neck). Many women delight in being able to go back to wearing low-lying crew necks or even V-neck shirts and sweaters, along with clavicle-flattering necklaces and chokers.

Recovery

After surgery, your face and head will be wrapped in bandages. You will likely be required to wear drains near the ears to catch the fluid that may leak from the incisions as your body starts to heal. After a day, your surgeon will remove these, along with the bandages. The incisions will be sensitive but shouldn't hurt. To minimize infection and pain, your doctor may prescribe antibiotics, an anti-inflammatory, and pain medication. Your stitches will either dissolve or need to be removed in about five days, depending on what type of sutures your doctor uses.

While you're healing, it is important to limit certain activities. Refrain from bending down or straining—or doing anything else that will bring blood to your face. Vigorous activity is out, including sex and housework, for at least two weeks (though walking and stretching are beneficial). Don't shower for a couple of days; plan on taking a lot of sponge baths. Sleep with your head elevated on at least two pillows. Avoid unneccessary phone calls (or use speakerphone), because holding a phone to your ear will be uncomfortable and potentially damaging to the sutures. Do not wear earrings for approximately six weeks. Since the ear is used to hide the incisions, any tension on the area—earrings catching on a sweater, say—could compromise healing. For the same reason, avoid pullover sweaters and shirts. You may go back to wearing makeup about seven days after surgery, so long as you avoid applying it near the sutured areas.

Common Side Effects

Tightness and/or Discomfort
Because of post-operative swelling, the area around the incisions may be sensitive. The discomfort is temporary and can be managed with pain medication. If

you feel outright pain, call your doctor immediately. At the end of the first week, I require all my surgery patients to have a lymphatic massage, a light-touch technique that helps the body heal by mobilizing the lymphatic fluids that contribute to swelling (for more on massage technique, see Chapter 12).

Blood and Fluid Drainage

This is easily managed with surgical drains that your doctor will likely insert at the incision sites. If you have what seem to be excessive amounts of fluid (more than the drains can handle), consult your doctor immediately.

Bruising and Swelling

Most bruising will be evident around the eyes and in the cheeks and neck. If you've had a neck lift, the bruising may even extend to the collarbone. (You may want to avoid mirrors for the first couple of days.) After two or three days, however, your normal color will reassert itself, and most bruising should fade within two weeks. Swelling in the face and neck is normal and can be controlled with anti-inflammatories supervised by your doctor.

Numbness

You may have some loss of sensation, especially around the cheeks, neck, and ears. Feeling may take several weeks, or even months, to return.

Scars and Scar Irritation

The incisions may feel itchy and uncomfortable as they heal. Scars should start to fade within two weeks, when you will probably feel okay about going outside, concealing them with makeup. Scars take several weeks to months to heal entirely.

Hair Loss

You may experience a thinning of hair near the incisions; this should grow back, except perhaps on the scars themselves.

SMOKERS' ALERT

Smoking is incredibly damaging to skin, especially on the face. It increases swelling and scarring, and impedes healing. Worst of all, because it cuts off blood flow to the skin's surface, smoking puts post-operative patients at risk for a complication called skin necrosis, where the skin dies rather than re-adheres, leaving a wound on the surface. Some physicians even refuse to perform face surgery on smokers. *At the very least, you must stop smoking two weeks before and not resume until at least two weeks after surgery.*

Side Effects to Be Concerned About

Facial Paralysis

Weakness or paralysis is the most significant, though rare, complication you may encounter (it happens in less than 1 percent of cases). It is possible during surgery for nerves to be cut or stretched, resulting in muscular paralysis and/or drooping in the eye or lip area. Should this occur, there can sometimes be a "sharing" of nerve function, where other nerves take over the job of a severed one, and sensation and movement are restored. But nerve damage is not something that is easily fixed in a follow-up.

Asymmetry

Every face starts off a bit uneven, and sometimes it isn't until after surgery that the asymmetry becomes apparent. But asymmetry may also result from damage to facial muscles or nerves during surgery, most likely in the smile or eyebrow area. This complication usually resolves itself over time. In the extremely unlikely event that it does not, however, a surgeon can perform a corrective procedure on the other side of the face to even it out.

Hairline Drift

When the skin around the ear is lifted and tucked, the edge of the hairline may recede slightly. A skilled surgeon can perform a corrective procedure if need be.

Keloid Scars

Most scars should flatten out and become less conspicuous within several weeks. In some people, however, scars become raised, red, and angry. This complication can be controlled with topical or injected steroids, pigment blockers, and laser and microdermabrasion treatments.

Hematoma

Blood pooling may occur within two days after surgery, and may be caused by elevated blood pressure due to excessive movement. To minimize risk, avoid vigorous activity or heavy lifting for the first few days postop.

Skin Death

If a patient smokes or has a hematoma, circulation to the skin is reduced, and small patches of skin on the face, especially around the ear, may die and/or fall off. These areas should eventually grow back on their own, though there may be a resulting scar.

Infection

If you experience significant pain, excessive swelling, and redness, or if you develop a fever, you may have an infection. While this is rare, it can be resolved with a cycle of antibiotics.

URGENT QUESTION: *IS IT BETTER TO HAVE LONG HAIR WHEN GETTING A FACE-LIFT?*

Long hair *does* provide more ways to conceal scars discreetly, especially those behind the ears, and may allow you to feel comfortable going out in public sooner than if you sport short hair. Long-haired patients who like to wear ponytails or up-dos, however, will have less success concealing the scars behind the ears. Conversely, those with short hair may opt for a fringy look in front of the ears to obscure the effects of their surgery. But the scars that run under the earlobe may be more visible, as well as those behind the hairline. Discuss these issues with your doctor; your hairstyle may affect where and how the doctor makes incisions.

THE GREAT FACE-LIFT ALTERNATIVE

So what do I do if *not* a traditional face-lift? I prefer a combination of smaller and less-invasive procedures, depending on a patient's particular grievances. If someone comes to me looking to have her or his whole face rejuvenated—the traditional face-lift candidate—typically I'll do an endoscopic forehead lift, an eyelid lift, and a mini-face-lift. If only the upper face is saggy or wrinkled, I may do just the forehead and eyes; if the lower half is most affected, I may go with simply a mini-lift.

While two or three procedures may not sound like a worthwhile trade-off for one, the fact is that these surgeries require smaller incisions, are less traumatic to the tissues, and have a quicker recovery than a traditional face-lift. What's more, the results are in my opinion superior: Because you aren't pulling all the tissues at once, in a single direction, the face looks more natural, or less "done." This is where the surgeon's artistry comes in. Looking at the planes of a patient's face, and his or her particular features, we vary our approach based on individual needs and desires. (I may even use fat injections or cheek or chin implants in conjunction with surgery to help create a balanced face.) We can now do less and less, sacrificing few, if any, of the benefits of a full face-lift. Following, I will go over each procedure in more detail.

MINI-FACE-LIFT OR "MINI-LIFT"
(MINI-RHYTIDECTOMY)

With a mini-lift, only the lower face—from cheek to chin—is lifted, which effectively eliminates jowls and redefines the cheekbones. As with a face-lift, the mini-lift is often accompanied by a neck lift, which removes fat from below the chin and tightens the neck's platysma muscles, all through a tiny incision under the chin. The best candidates for the mini-lift are those who are unhappy with the contour of their lower face and neck, and whose skin has good resiliency. It's also an ideal procedure for a patient who is somewhat gun-shy about going all the way with a major overhaul.

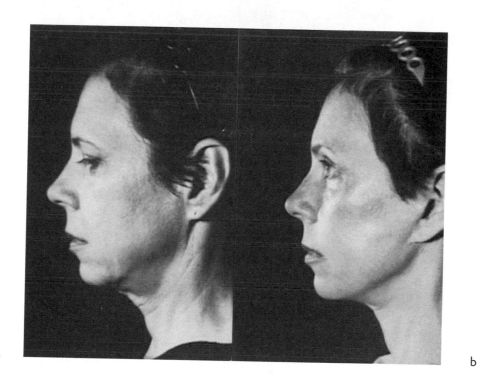

a   b

A POPULAR COMBO: MINI-LIFT, ENDOSCOPIC FOREHEAD LIFT, AND EYELID LIFT

While this forty-nine-year-old patient's neck and jowl area are most visibly sagging (a), I felt that to do only a mini-lift on the lower face would leave the upper face looking old and out of sync. So we decided also to do an endoscopic forehead lift and eyelid lift, which raised her eyebrows, opened her eyes, and got rid of the fullness around the lids (b). At the same time I injected some fat into her lips, which had thinned with age, and her nasolabial folds, to get rid of some of the age-related flattening. She's happy she took care of everything in one surgery rather than two.

Take Martha, the sixty-four-year-old volunteer worker whose story I recounted earlier. "I was not a person who felt comfortable with the idea of surgery," she recalls. "In fact, I was always enormously critical of other people who chose it. I have friends who had a lift ten, even five years ago, and they just all look so 'pulled.' I knew I didn't want to come out looking that way." Martha was particularly worried that she would be "found out"; I assured her that with a mini-lift, the effects would be so subtle—the eyes, for example, are left alone and can't possibly become stretched in that catlike way—that people would merely think she'd been on a restorative vacation. Martha's experience supported this:

> *"A couple of weeks after my surgery, I attended a big charity luncheon and met several women I hadn't seen in a while. They all told me I looked great; some even asked if I'd changed my hair or lost weight (actually, I'd gained a little!). Honestly, I look ten years younger."*

Tanya was another perfect candidate for a mini-lift. "I was losing definition in my jawline, and over the years the skin on my neck had grown crepey," recalls the fifty-one-year-old schoolteacher. "The lines on either side of my chin, what I call my 'puppet' lines, were getting deeper, too." Her upper face was fine, however: She had very little sun damage or puffiness near her eyes, and little wrinkling on her forehead. Because we needed only to tighten her face from the cheekbones down, we elected to do a mini-lift. Tanya's results were subtle, but made a world of difference. "My husband had felt the surgery was totally unnecessary, but supported me in my decision," Tanya continues. "A couple of weeks after the operation, when I hadn't completely healed and started to worry, I turned to him for reassurance. He scrutinized my face for a minute, and said, 'You know, I haven't really looked at you closely in twenty-five years.' For a moment, my heart sank. But what a change! From that moment on, he's been looking at me through new eyes. He thinks I look terrific."

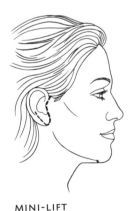

MINI-LIFT

What the Surgery Involves

The mini-lift patient is usually under twilight sedation and a local anesthetic. The incision starts at the top of the ear, rather than at the temple as in a traditional lift. It runs in front of the ear and behind the little bump of cartilage called the tragus, and ends just behind the earlobe without running back into the scalp, see illustration. The skin is then separated from the fat and underlying muscle; the fat and muscle are recontoured and all layers are pulled tight; the excess skin is removed; and the incision is sutured with dissolvable or regular sutures. If the neck needs work, your doctor may also make a tiny incision under the chin and use liposuction to suck out the fat, then tighten the platysma muscles in the neck. The whole process typically takes three to four hours.

Recovery

When you wake up, your face will be wrapped in a loose dressing that helps to hold the skin in place. These bandages stay on for twenty-four hours; you may have drains placed near the incisions to catch any fluid that results from healing. You'll probably have some localized soreness, too, but your doctor will prescribe anti-inflammatory and pain medication for the swelling and discomfort, as well as an antibiotic to reduce the risk of infection. If you experience severe pain once you get home, that isn't normal, and you should notify your doctor immediately. The following day, your surgeon will remove the dressing (perhaps replacing it with a lighter one). Stitches will dissolve or will require removal in about five days, depending on the type of sutures used.

Recovery experiences are individual. Here are the recollections of Leslie, a fifty-nine-year-old attorney who had a mini-lift along with a nose and eye job:

"The first two days were really crummy. Because of my nose, I couldn't wear my glasses, so everything was out of focus. My face was numb and uncomfortable. When I got my bandages off and saw the puffiness, I thought, 'Oh my God, what have I done?' For a few days you worry that you'll never be yourself again.

"Of course, you are, eventually. After nearly two weeks I went back to work. I was still slightly bruised, a little brown and green, but I wore concealing makeup and I really think that no one could tell unless they were studying my face. Five weeks after surgery, I went to a wedding shower for my daughter, and I was totally comfortable facing people. Two months later, I felt wonderful, more confident, and so happy to look and feel young again. And one other thing: For the last fifteen years or so I'd worn my hair short, which just seemed appropriate for a woman my age. After the surgery, though, I grew it long again, the way I used to wear it years ago."

Just as often, however, my patients report that recovery from a mini-face-lift is quite manageable. Says Patricia:

> *"Afterward I kind of looked like Hannibal Lecter with my bandaged and bruised face. But I wasn't in any real pain. I had the surgery on a Thursday, and on Monday I went out to the movies. A week later, because I didn't have much bruising on my face, I even went to a restaurant with friends whom I didn't tell about the surgery."*

The symptoms to expect after surgery are very similar to those for the traditional face-lift. The main difference is that bruising will start in the midface; the eyes should be pretty much unaffected. Because the incisions are shorter than in a full face-lift, the healing process will be a little quicker, with less visible swelling and scarring.

The attendant risks of a mini-lift are the same as for a face-lift; these include infection, asymmetry, hematoma, and in very rare cases, severed nerves.

ENDOSCOPIC FOREHEAD (OR "BROW") LIFT

Endoscopy is largely responsible for the transformation of the face-lift business—not to mention medicine in general. When the magnificent fiber-optic instrument known as an endoscope is used on almost any area of the body, a major operation requiring large incisions suddenly becomes a minor one, requiring only tiny slits.

An endoscope is a tube-shaped probe with a tiny light and miniature video camera on one end. When I insert the endoscope through an incision (which I make as small as a quarter-inch), I can see what's going on underneath the skin and view the proceedings on a TV monitor in the operating room. The video allows me to rely on both touch and sight to perform robotlike surgery, in which I maneuver the endoscope with one hand and surgical instruments with the other.

I most commonly use this instrument to perform an endoscopic forehead

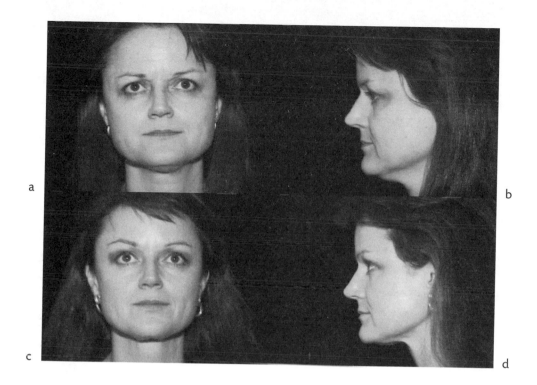

a

b

c

d

ENDOSCOPIC FOREHEAD LIFT

The best way to get rid of that "angry" look (a, b)? An endoscopic forehead lift. This forty-six-year-old business executive came to me seeking an eyelid lift, but I thought I could get better results by lifting the entire brow. With only three tiny incisions in her hairline, I lifted the whole forehead, which opened her eyes, eliminated the furrow between her brows, and brightened the upper face all the way down to her cheekbones (c, d).

or brow lift, which opens and brightens the upper face, smooths deep furrows and wrinkles in the forehead, softens the vertical scowl lines between the eyebrows, lifts sagging brows, alleviates pressure on the upper eyelid, and even lifts the nose a bit. Because drooping brows and forehead furrows are such evident markers of age and stress as early as one's mid-thirties, this procedure is among the most popular I perform. For me, it has thoroughly supplanted the more traditional forehead or brow lift, which I haven't done in years and can't imagine ever doing again. With a traditional lift, the incision runs across the top of the head, from one ear to the other, see illustration on page 122. The more prominent scarring, bruising, and swelling mean a longer recovery; there's a greater chance of numbness in the scalp; and, not infrequently, the eyebrows are too high, resulting in a permanent startled look. Of course, there are patients and doctors out there who prefer the tighter appearance that a traditional forehead lift provides, and some do it with very pleasing results.

FOREHEAD LIFT BONUS: MIGRAINE RELIEF

Patients who get a traditional or endoscopic forehead lift may experience a surprising and beneficial side effect: the alleviation of migraine headaches. According to a recent study, 80 percent of those with migraines who underwent a forehead lift were either cured completely or experienced significant relief. Some experts think the key to the migraine cure is the removal of the "corrugator muscles" located between the eyebrows, which may short-circuit the neural transference of pain messages.

What the Surgery Involves

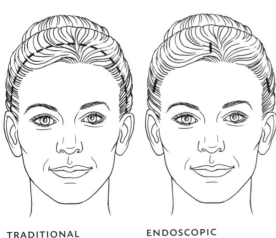

TRADITIONAL
FOREHEAD LIFT

ENDOSCOPIC
FOREHEAD LIFT

With the patient under twilight sedation and local anesthesia, the surgeon makes a couple of small incisions—generally three, each under a half-inch, just behind the hairline, see illustration at right. Unlike a traditional brow lift, an endoscopic lift does not require that any hair be removed. Although small, the incisions are deep and penetrate to the skull, so the underlying tissue, muscle, and skin can be separated from the bone to which they're attached. The doctor will also cut some muscle—

the ones that cause the cleft between the eyes, called the "corrugator" muscles—and detach the eyebrows from the orbital bone. The skin and muscle are then lifted, so that the saggy brow and deep forehead wrinkles are eliminated or improved. Temporary sutures secure the skin in its new, higher position. While it heals, the skin adheres to the face's deeper tissue. The surgery takes roughly one hour.

Recovery

The post-op feeling is generally not painful, just uncomfortable. You may feel a little tightening around the forehead; some people say it can be a bit claustrophobic. You may also have some short-term numbness at the incision sites or just behind them. Your doctor will probably prescribe an anti-inflammatory medication and painkillers for potential discomfort, and an antibiotic to prevent infection. You'll need to keep a surgical dressing around your head for a few days as the incisions heal. (I advocate also wearing a surgical band for a day or two to hold the forehead in position.) Don't jump when you look in the mirror and your brow looks as if it's drifting up to your hairline: Usually a surgeon "overcorrects" the forehead—that is, lifts the eyebrows *above* where they're ultimately going to settle—so the skin doesn't adhere too low.

Common Side Effects

Discomfort
Tightening is likely to occur around the crown of the head, though there should be no outright pain.

Bruising
The skin is detached from the underlying bone and redraped, so some internal bleeding and skin discoloration will occur, especially around the eyes. Because the incisions are in the scalp, however, you can wear makeup before they heal entirely to cover up the bruised areas.

Numbness

There may be some loss of sensation around the forehead and eyes, which usually clears up within several weeks but may take up to several months. There may also be numbness in the skin around the scars.

Contour Irregularities

You may find you have a small bump of extra skin behind the ear. That's normal, and it diminishes over several weeks, or sometimes months, as the skin redistributes itself and evens out.

Side Effects to Be Concerned About

Nerve Damage

Though it is unlikely, nerves may be stretched during surgery, resulting in weakness of the eyelids or eyebrows that can last several weeks to several months. In 3 percent of all instances, the nerves are severed and the damage is permanent.

Raised Hairline

Because the skin is being pulled, the surgery may cause the hairline to recede slightly.

Hematoma

A temporary accumulation of blood under the skin may slow healing, but it should clear up within a couple of days.

Hair Loss

You may have very small bald patches near the scars. In severe cases, the area can be excised and closed up to repair the condition.

Infection

If you experience excessive pain and redness, or if you come down with a fever, you may have an infection. While this is very rare, it is easily cured with antibiotics. See your doctor immediately.

NECK LIFT AND NECK LIPECTOMY

A saggy, fatty "gobble neck" can add more years to a face than a whole head of gray hair. "I was thin and in good shape," recalls Beth, a fifty-four-year-old book publisher, "but my neck just dragged down my whole appearance." The neck lift is an easy way to reduce jowls, eliminate a double chin, slim the bands of muscle that form the wattle (recently, and oddly, celebrated as an erogenous zone on TV's *Ally McBeal*), and tighten neck skin. Like the endoscopic forehead lift and mini-face-lift, the neck lift also delivers highly satisfying results with a minimum of physical and psychological trauma. (I often do the procedure on a Thursday, to have patients back at work on Monday.) Typically, a surgeon will also decide to perform a lipectomy, suctioning out fat in order to resculpt the area; she or he may insert a chin implant to create even more definition.

What the Surgery Involves

The surgery is typically done under twilight sedation with local anesthesia. A lipectomy is performed through an incision less than a centimeter long (about one-third of an inch) under the chin and a two-millimeter incision in the crease of the earlobe. A cannula is inserted through each hole, and fat is liposuctioned out in order to resculpt the neckline.

The very act of liposuction stimulates the skin to tighten, and the muscles may now be cut and recontoured. If a neck lift is also being performed, excess skin will be removed. To do that, the surgeon makes an incision at some distance from the neck, typically around the ear, lifts the skin and some of the tissues underneath, and sutures it into position.

Both procedures take one to two hours.

Recovery

The post-op feeling is typically not painful, just uncomfortable. You will likely get an anti-inflammatory medication and painkiller for potential dis-

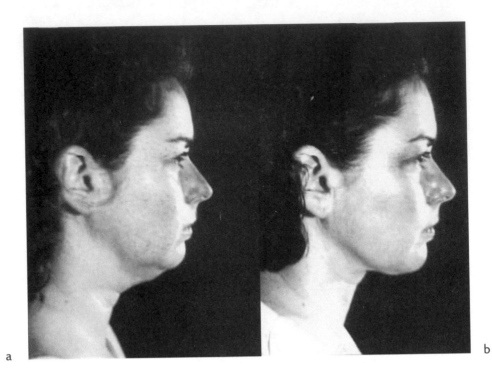

NECK LIPECTOMY

A "gobble neck" can now be sucked away in just a few minutes with a neck lipectomy. This forty-four-year-old lawyer had a hereditary fullness in the neck that had grown worse with age (a). I suctioned out the fat through a tiny hole under her chin, then tightened the underlying neck muscles through the same incision. Look how dramatically different the "after" picture (b) is!

comfort, and an antibiotic to diminish the risk of infection. While every patient must wear a neck dressing for one to two days, normal head movement is encouraged, as it helps the healing process by allowing the skin to stretch to its normal limits. Don't exercise vigorously for at least two weeks, though: Raising your blood pressure can increase the risk of hematoma. You may experience some numbness in the whole neck region, particularly around the scars.

All in all, I find neck lifts and lipectomies to be terrific surgeries for many people. They can tighten the neck and lower face through a tiny incision, yielding results comparable to those of some face-lifts.

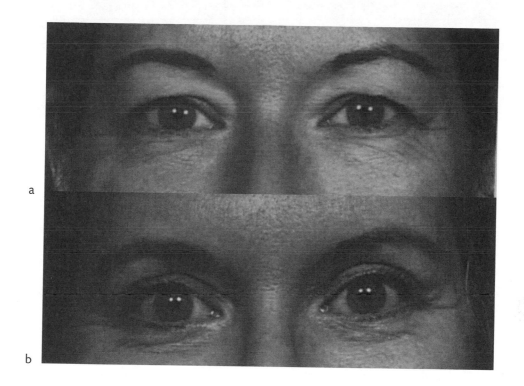

a

b

EYELID LIFT

This otherwise-youthful forty-three-year-old teacher's hooded lids made her look sleepy (a). Through an imperceptible incision in the crease, I performed a blepharoplasty, removing the extra skin and fatty pockets in her upper lids. Today her eyes are much brighter and more youthful looking (b).

EYELID SURGERY
(BLEPHAROPLASTY OR "EYELID LIFT")

The eyes, windows to the soul, too often seem to reveal exhaustion. The very delicate skin around the eyes gets crepey and puffy from fatigue and stress, and eyelid surgery has become one of the most popular procedures I do. In fact, it's not uncommon for someone to appear otherwise young and healthy, but have eyes that tell a different story.

Remember Jim, the forty-six-year-old computer executive who had the

Light-Bulb Moment about getting surgery in Chapter 1? His eyelids, the right one in particular, sagged so much that co-workers routinely ribbed him about looking as if he'd been out partying all night, and he felt it was affecting his standing in the company. "In my business, first impressions mean a lot, and I was worried about the message my appearance was sending to clients," he says. Cutting back on his hours might have helped the appearance of his eyes. However, not all eye puffiness is the result of overwork, inadequate sleep, or other lifestyle factors. Some people are born with hooded lids caused by excess skin that sometimes impairs vision; others have fatty deposits above or below the eye, or both.

In Jim's case, I performed a blepharoplasty on both his upper and lower eyelids so his look would be consistent, top and bottom. The puffiness and circles are gone, and his eyes are as open and bright as if he'd awoken from a weeklong nap. He now feels more optimistic about his professional outlook, knowing he benefits both from his years of experience and his once-again youthful demeanor.

Eyelid surgery has evolved considerably over the years. Incisions are so small that they leave no trace of a scar. In the past, we might have removed fat from around the eye, but the patient was often left with a haunted, hollowed-out look. Now, for better results, we often just reposition the fat, since it holds up the skin. And by doing an endoscopic forehead lift along with eyelid surgery, we can achieve even better results. Blepharoplasty is a common procedure, costs less than many others, and should bring immediate and dramatic improvement.

What the Surgery Involves

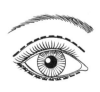
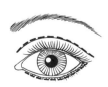

EYELID LIFT

Eyelid lifts are typically done using twilight sedation and a local anesthetic. The surgeon makes an incision along the lower lashes that will be almost invisible when it heals, see illustration, then either removes fat or, more likely, redistributes it. The saggy and crepey

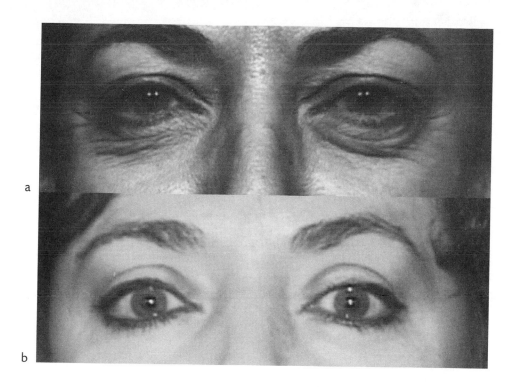

a

b

EYELID LIFT WITH ENDOSCOPIC FOREHEAD LIFT

Sometimes, to get rid of puffy eyes *and* a droopy brow (a), I'll perform an eyelid lift and endoscopic forehead lift simultaneously. This fifty-five-year-old advertising executive had both, and appears much younger and more alert after the procedure (b).

excess skin is then pulled up and cut off. The incision is closed with tiny sutures, which are removed in four to six days.

If excess upper eyelid skin is hooding the eye and needs to be eliminated, an incision is made about ten millimeters above the eyelashes in the palpebral fold, the crease at the top of the lid, see illustration at left on page 128, and excess skin and fat are removed. The incisions are closed and sutured on the underside of the skin. A blepharoplasty takes forty-five minutes to an hour.

Recovery

Although you may receive only a mild sedative during surgery, the ointment in your eyes (administered to help prevent infection and minimize swelling) may blur your vision upon waking and you'll need someone to take you home. After three days you'll no longer need the ointment, but contact lenses are forbidden for another couple of weeks. To help minimize bruising, keep your head up: Even hunching over a book can cause fluid to pool, and lead to discoloration and puffiness. Since the skin around the eyes is delicate, an eyelid lift carries a greater risk of bruising than some other facial procedures, so plan on wearing dark sunglasses for a few days and taking off at least one week from work. You may also find that the eyes don't close completely for a few days; drops can ease the dryness.

"The stitches were uncomfortable, and I was black and blue around the eyes," recalls Jim, "but the recovery moved along pretty quickly. By the time I went back to work one week later, I had traces of a black eye, but if anybody noticed it, they didn't say anything."

A FASTER FIX FOR THE EYES

When all you have is puffiness around the eye, but no sagging, it's possible to reduce the puffiness from the inside, with almost no recovery time, using a *subconjunctival blepharoplasty*. I recently performed one on a fashion model on a Thursday, and she did a photo shoot the following Monday. Fat is excised from inside the eyelid using a scalpel; then the area is cauterized to stop the bleeding. Since the incision is out of sight, there will be no trace of the surgery, except for maybe a tiny bit of bruising that can easily be concealed with makeup. This procedure heals in a week, and is a great quick fix.

CHIN AUGMENTATION (MENTOPLASTY)

A weak chin causes legions to curse their fate, grow beards that become lifetime disguises, wear concealing scarves and turtlenecks, and try to avoid being

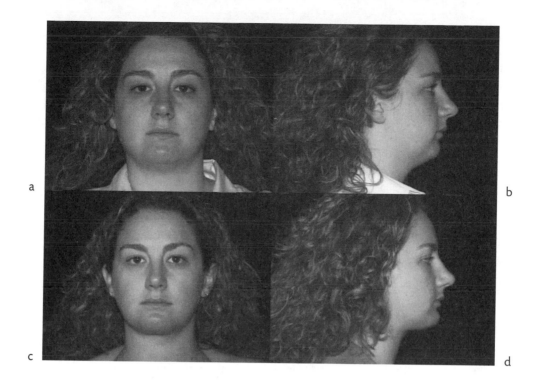

a

b

c

d

NECK LIPECTOMY WITH CHIN AUGMENTATION

This twenty-six-year-old patient has a trim figure, but her neck, exacerbated by her receding chin, made her look chubby (a, b). I did a neck lipectomy to suction out the fat and tighten the underlying muscles, and added a chin implant to help give her jaw area more definition. Today she not only looks thinner, but the entire contour of her face has changed (c, d).

---

viewed in profile. A mentoplasty to improve a weak chin can work wonders. An artful surgeon not only will make the chin more prominent, but will do so in a way that better complements the nose (among other anatomical landmarks) and improves the face's overall symmetry and harmony. The maxilla and mandible—the upper and lower parts of the jaw—will also be better aligned by a chin implant. It's rare that I do chin augmentation without also doing a necklift or neck lipectomy, which eliminates jowls and slims a wattle.

What the Surgery Involves

Chin augmentation is usually done using twilight sedation and local anesthesia. The surgeon makes an incision either inside the mouth, where there will be no visible scarring, or under the chin in the area's natural crease. An implant is inserted above the chin bone, where it is secured with sutures (my preference) or a screw. The chin-shaped implant comes in a variety of compositions. Some are porous, others not; some are made of polymers, and some of silicone. New implant materials are continually being developed as we strive for the most natural look possible. Scar tissue will form around the implant, helping to keep it in place. A pressure bandage helps, too, which patients wear for two to three days. Chin augmentation typically takes one to two hours.

Recovery

You will be up and around immediately after this procedure, but because the implant can shift for the first four to six weeks following surgery, you must avoid vigorous activity that could dislodge it, especially contact sports or those where you risk getting beaned by a ball. In very rare cases the implant can adhere out of position, which requires follow-up surgery to correct. Keep your head elevated and apply ice to reduce swelling. Brushing teeth and chewing may be tough for a week or so, as will smiling and even talking (you may want to wait a week to commit to any public speaking engagements). There may also be some numbness around the implant area or lips, but this sensation should go away within a couple of weeks.

CHEEK IMPLANTS

The aging of the midface—below the eyes and above the mouth—profoundly affects the face's overall look. When the cheeks start to droop, a person tends to appear older and chronically tired, which may be why many older women cake on such heavy rouge to create definition. For someone who has lost volume in the cheek area with age, implants can create higher cheekbones, lift the skin, and give the face a youthful plumpness and brightness. They are also flattering for younger patients who have a very round face and flat cheeks, or a narrow face that lacks definition.

An alternative to inserting implants is to use one's own fat to augment or enhance the cheeks. This autologous fat is typically retrieved from the thighs, hips, buttocks, or stomach. Implants may be used in conjunction with a mini-lift or alone. (One popular combo is to implant fat around the lips and nasolabial folds.)

What the Surgery Involves

During surgery, a small incision is made inside the mouth in the buccal sulcus, the crease where the upper lip meets the gums above the teeth, and triangular silicone implants are inserted through the opening and moved to the cheek area. Once in place, the implant overlies the bone, where it's sutured in. If autologous fat, rather than implants, is being used to plump up the midface, then it may also be inserted through this crease.

Recovery

When you first look in the mirror, you'll probably be suffering from a bad case of chipmunk cheeks. Be patient about seeing the result you desire; the immediate swelling and bruising will last a week or two. Some basic activities like eating, talking, and brushing teeth may be uncomfortable during that time. Complications with this surgery are rare. As with all procedures, for several weeks you should avoid vigorous exercise, which can dislodge implants and raise blood pressure, raising the risk of hematoma.

EAR SURGERY (OTOPLASTY)

"Dumbo" or "jug" ears—ears that stick out—are easily fixed, as are excessively large earlobes. Because overly prominent ears are something one is born with, we try to correct the problem in children just before they begin schooling, when they're sure to be taunted for their looks. By age eight, ears reach 80 percent of their adult growth. Many adults with cosmetic ear problems who come to see me didn't have access to corrective surgery when they were young, but those years of feeling self-conscious needn't continue. We can easily rectify the problem at any age. Insurance may even cover the procedure, because the condition, if extreme, is considered a deformity.

What the Surgery Involves

Otoplasty is a quick operation done under twilight sedation and local anesthesia. Three- to four-inch incisions are made behind the ear, and ear cartilage is cut and repositioned closer to the head with stitches (cartilage has "memory" and will want to return to its previous position unless it is sutured). Excess skin may be removed, and the incisions stitched back up. The procedure lasts about an hour and a half (forty-five minutes per ear).

Recovery

Patients are required to wear a headband for a week after surgery and for up to six weeks at night, to make sure the cartilage re-adheres correctly. The post-op feeling is generally not painful, just uncomfortable, and your doctor will typically administer anti-inflammatory medication and a painkiller for the swelling and potential discomfort. Vigorous exercise is forbidden for two weeks so that healing isn't interrupted and to minimize the chance of hematoma. Talking on the phone (unless you use a speakerphone) should be avoided for at least three days. If, over time, the ears don't hold their new position exactly, another surgery—equally quick and easy—can rectify this.

NOSE JOB (RHINOPLASTY)

The nose is an extension of the face, the first thing one sees—but not the first thing one should notice. That honor goes to the eyes. If a nose is out of proportion with the midface, we can correct this and return attention to the eyes.

The cosmetic nose problems we most commonly correct are an unsightly or crooked hump (dorsum), a nose sagging from age, and a bulbous or shapeless tip that needs refining. Since the nose is a functional entity as well, certain mechanical and structural problems—breathing difficulties, perpetual stuffiness, deviated septum, and post-nasal drip, among others—can also be corrected with a nose job.

Hesitancy about getting rhinoplasty is fading fast thanks to developments of the last fifteen years, particularly aesthetic ones. It used to be, of course, that all nose-job noses were transparently unnatural: straight, upturned, pinched, and minuscule. Old-school Dr. X would give all his patients the unmistakably signature Dr. X nose. But over the years, tastes have shifted. Surgeons started doing less rather than more, displaying a welcome sense of restraint and refinement in crafting a more natural-looking nose.

Today, we look at the shape of the candidate's face, the width of the cheeks, the position of the eyes and the distance between them, the thickness of the skin, and the candidate's ethnic background. With all that to consider, we can then determine what nose size and shape would be most proportional and appealing. Computer imaging, as you might guess, has been profoundly helpful. Doctor and patient together visualize the new nose; in determining how much to reduce a hump, for instance, I can actually alter the percentage of its reduction by single degrees until a patient says to me, "Okay, I like it there." Lots of men want to leave at least a little hump in their nose. With computer imaging, they can show me exactly how much.

In our pursuit of a more natural nose, a procedure (one that I've never embraced) called an "open rhinoplasty" came into vogue a few years ago. Practitioners thought they had more control over a subject's nose if they could see into it, so they made an incision below the tip, opened up the nose, and reconstructed the cartilage. To leave a scar in a prominent position that's not absolutely necessary makes no sense to me. I prefer to operate while the

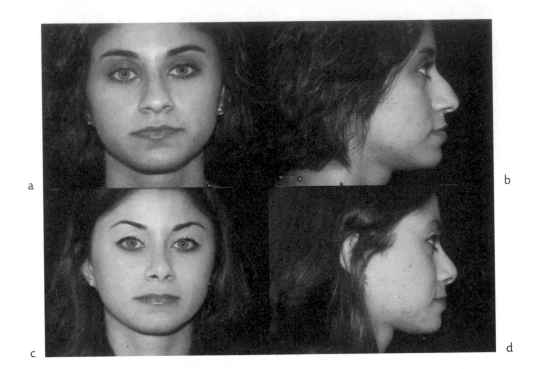

RHINOPLASTY: FLATTENING, NARROWING THE BRIDGE

This twenty-four-year-old Iranian patient wanted me to soften the bump in her nose, and narrow the bridge (a, b). I am wary of taking a nose job too far, and feared that a small, turned-up nose wouldn't be harmonious with her wide face and large eyes. Instead, we opted for a straight nose that is only very slightly turned up at the tip (all surgery was done from the inside of her nose, so there's no scar). She went from lacking confidence in her appearance to looking quite glamorous (c, d).

nose is "closed" and make my incisions on the inside of the nose, thus concealing the evidence of my work. So ask your surgeon whether he or she performs an "open" or "closed" nose job, and about the advantages and disadvantages of each for your particular case.

Another positive development: Unlike a generation ago, when surgeons performing nose jobs only reduced, now we sometimes *add,* to improve the nose both structurally and aesthetically. We may add bone (taken from the skull, hip, or rib cage) or cartilage (taken from the nose or ear), or a synthetic material like silicone or Goretex, to build it up, as there may not be enough underneath to work with.

AVOID CARBON-COPY NOSES

A nose should fit your facial features, skin tone, ethnicity, and even height, and a good surgeon will work with you to arrive at the optimally harmonious look. But many surgeons have a favorite style: the ski jump, the pug, the narrow bridge, etc. When interviewing doctors, be sure to ask to see their work. Have them show you photographs or computer images, or even point out any nurses or other staff who have had a nose job done by them. If you see that each nose is an exact replica of the next, be wary: You want a nose that pleases *you*, not just your surgeon.

URGENT QUESTION:
WILL INSURANCE COVER MY RHINOPLASTY?

Unfortunately, fewer and fewer plastic surgery procedures are covered by insurance, even when they correct a functional problem. However, I've known insurers to cover surgery to alleviate breathing difficulties, either because of a deviated septum or swelling of the hypertrophic turbinates (structures inside the nose that help fight off infection). The prevention of snoring is also covered when there's a medical reason to correct it (for instance, if it's linked to sleep apnea). Reconstruction of a broken nose is reimbursed under most medical plans, too. But there's a lot of paperwork for both you and your doctor to complete, as wary insurers treat cosmetic procedures with heightened suspicion. Talk to your doctor about coverage before proceeding.

"My nose was wide at the end, and protruded from my face more than I would have liked. It was so out of proportion, and as I got older, I got more self-conscious about it. It became like this invisible weight I was carrying around. I first started thinking about a nose job in college, but I didn't know anyone who'd had plastic surgery, and I didn't have the guts or, frankly, the money. But when I got out of college, I thought, 'I don't want to spend my twenties in hiding. I want to feel I can go anywhere and be comfortable with myself.' That's what gave me the motivation to finally do something about it, and I'm so glad that I did."

—Alison, 23, accountant

What the Surgery Involves

During rhinoplasty you're under twilight sedation, numbed by a local anesthetic. In the case of a "closed" rhinoplasty the surgeon will work exclusively inside the nose, using a headlight and magnifying glasses. He or she will shave the dorsum (the top of the nose) and break the bones on either side of it for repositioning. To shape the tip, cartilage is either removed or molded. Once the changes are in place, the incisions are sutured—again, from inside the nose. (If nostrils are being reduced in size, there will be a small scar on the outside of the nose.) If you're having an "open" rhinoplasty, an incision will be made in the skin between the nostrils, and the skin and underlying tissues lifted like a tent so the surgeon can move the bone and cartilage.

Recovery

Since bone is broken in this procedure, it's likely you'll come out resembling a prizefighter after the tenth round. I simply tell patients to avoid looking in the mirror for a few days. A lightweight cast is applied to the top of the nose to

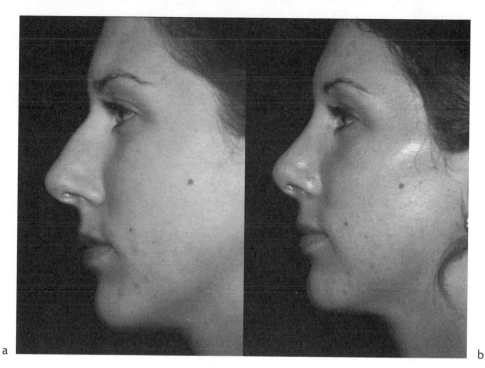

a

b

RHINOPLASTY: SMOOTHING THE BUMP, SOFTENING THE TIP

This twenty-four-year-old securities broker inherited delicate Irish features. As a result, her nose, which projected out quite far, was the first thing you saw when you looked at her (a). We decided her face could handle a bit of a turned-up sweep, and so I did a nose job, softening the tip and smoothing out the bump (b). The result is a nose that is slightly less prominent, but still well in proportion.

keep the cartilage and bone in place during healing, and gauze packing is inserted in the nose for one to two days to protect the septum from moving and to minimize bleeding. While I've known a few patients who have felt perfectly comfortable dining out at restaurants when wearing the cast, most people go into hiding for a few days while the bruising and swelling subside.

The post-op feeling is generally not painful, just uncomfortable; your doctor will probably give you anti-inflammatory medication and a painkiller for swelling and discomfort, as well as an antibiotic to prevent infection. For the first twenty-four hours, apply ice and elevate the head on a couple of pil-

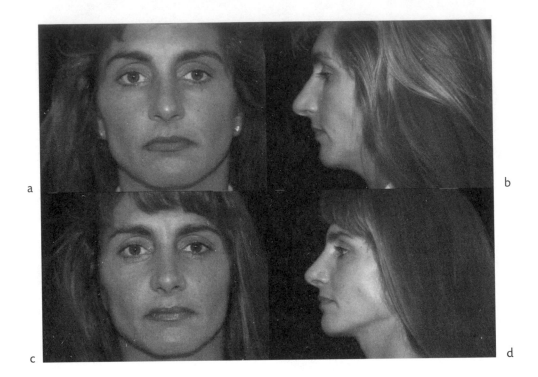

a

b

c

d

RHINOPLASTY: CHANGING THE ANGLE

This thirty-six-year-old always hated the look of her nose, believing that it stuck out too far from her face (a, b). I shortened the tip and, because the space between her nose and lip is so short, turned it up just a touch. The effect is a dramatic brightening of her entire face (c, d)!

lows (you can move around, but be conservative). At first, you may have difficulty breathing through the nose. Avoid blowing your nose, wearing eyeglasses, or otherwise jostling the cast.

After a week, the cast comes off. Despite the swelling and bruising, the results are immediate. Alison recalls: "I'll never forget the day the cast was removed: My face was yellow, my lips were numb, I could barely move my mouth, but there was my nose—narrower and elegant. I loved it the first time I saw it."

Common Side Effects

Throbbing and/or Discomfort

You should not experience outright pain, but there will be moderate discomfort for the first couple of days until swelling begins to subside—more if nasal bones are broken in the procedure.

Swelling

To minimize swelling inside the nose, which can last for weeks, your doctor may prescribe a nasal steroid spray. For outside, icing every twenty minutes or so helps; keep your head elevated for the first two days.

Bruising

Black eyes are a common side effect and should resolve within one to two weeks.

Congestion

Swollen tissues may make it tough to breathe for a couple of days. Congestion may also temporarily affect your sense of smell and taste. Using a humidifier may help keep nasal passages moist and encourage the incision to heal faster. Your doctor may also prescribe a decongestant to help clear things up.

Bleeding

This may occur for three to four days after the operation; call the doctor if it seems excessive or continues beyond this time.

Temporary Numbness

You may feel this especially around the tip of the nose and mouth; the condition should clear up on its own within a couple of weeks.

Side Effects to Be Concerned About

Serious complications are rare after rhinoplasty. A few things to watch out for:

Breathing Difficulties
If after several weeks you are still having trouble breathing, it may be due to scarring inside the nose. Consult your surgeon.

Sinus Infection
Swelling may block the nasal passage, triggering sinusitis. Telltale signs include thick mucous, severe headaches (especially near the eyes), and fevers. Call your doctor if you experience any of these.

Hematoma
Blood can pool beneath the skin, which can be triggered by exercise, vigorous activity, or high blood pressure.

Damaged Tear Ducts
You may experience increased (or dramatic reduction in) tearing, but this is very rare.

Malformed Shape
If the tissues do not heal correctly, or if your surgeon removes too much cartilage, the tip may collapse or look pinched. If a disproportionate amount of bone and cartilage is removed from the bridge, the result will be a ski-jump look. Both unfortunate problems are fixable with a follow-up procedure.

QUOTE, UNQUOTE

" I work with racehorses. I'd had a bump on my nose forever, which was made worse by getting kicked in the face by a horse. I had been insecure about my appearance my whole life. At first, I didn't have the money to do anything about it; later, I didn't have the courage. I'm a regularly attractive person, I've never had a problem dating or anything, but every once in a while someone would remark on my nose. I hated looking in the mirror so much that I never did. I never even put makeup on, my self-esteem was so low.

"Then a friend of mine had a nose job, and I thought she looked great. So I signed on for mine. All the work was done from the inside. During the operation, we discovered I had a deviated septum. I'd suffered headaches my whole life that were so bad, there were times I couldn't go to work. The doctor told me she could fix that and straighten out my nose, too. The recovery wasn't bad—I took nine days off from work and didn't ride a horse for a month. When I went back for a visit after one month and saw on the computer my 'before' and 'after,' the transformation was so startling I couldn't believe it. I have very petite features, and my nose is much more in scale with the rest of them. My face has gained some fullness and you don't just concentrate on what's in the middle. And one of the best things about the surgery is that it cut down my headaches by about 99 percent. I feel as if I've been hiding behind a wall my whole life, and didn't realize until now how much my looks had held me back."

—Lydia, 36, horse trainer

9

Breasts:
Size Matters

We women are incredibly aware of our breast appearance—maybe even more than *men* are. Breasts are sexual and sensual, a big part of what make us women, and they can dictate our sense of attractiveness and desirability (for better or worse).

Beautiful breasts needn't be just the privilege of youth. I see many women who have had issues about their breasts for years, even decades. What finally brought them to a decision point—that Light-Bulb Moment? Maybe child-bearing and breastfeeding left them hanging, so to speak. Or they could no longer tolerate the back pain caused by extra-large breasts. Or a life change—a new relationship, say, or an empty nest—provided the freedom and the guts to jump from a B to the C-plus cup they'd always secretly coveted. A couple of years ago, I performed a breast implant and lift on an eighty-year-old French woman who wished to sunbathe topless in her native country—with excellent results. For growing numbers of women, one of the biggest factors is critical mass (figuratively, not literally): Many more women are having breast surgery and talking about it openly, furthering the perception that procedures, and therefore results, are getting better all the time.

What determines the size of your breasts? A combination of genetics and, to an extent, weight. Breasts are composed of glandular or mammary tissue and some fat. Unfortunately, you can't shrink your breasts substantially through diet. But the presence of fat *does* give doctors more options for shaping them. In just the last couple of years, liposuction, requiring only the tiniest incision under the breast, has become a popular reduction method.

The best thing about breast surgery, be it augmentation, lift, or reduction, is that it's relatively painless and the recovery is quick. And since any immediate bruising or scarring is hidden by clothing, patients don't have to miss more than a few days of work.

You may never have 100-percent perfect, "Baywatch-babe" breasts. But you *can* have bigger ones, smaller ones, perkier ones, or fuller ones, potentially removing a long-standing obstacle to higher self-esteem, with minimal to-do. In the aftermath of her divorce, one of my patients, a woman in her early forties, decided to get a simple uplift to boost her spirits—and did it ever! On one of her first dates as a single woman post-surgery, she worked up the courage to wear a low-cut dress. At one point, her companion actually leaned across the table and confessed that he couldn't help admiring them. With so many other things in life causing stress or pain, or just emotional discomfort, your breasts should not be one of them.

GETTING BIGGER: IMPLANTS

Remember the old Clairol slogan about hair coloring, "Does she . . . or doesn't she?" That's the same question people ask themselves about breast implants, which can now look so natural as to be virtually undetectable. Breast augmentation is one of the top three most popular plastic surgery procedures performed. In the year 2001, more than 216,000 women in the United States had breast augmentation (formal name: *augmentation mammoplasty*), a 114 percent increase since 1997. So many women embrace this procedure because it carries little risk of complication. And because an implant can be inserted through a tiny incision in the navel or armpit (and moved into place under the skin), or under the areola or breast, it's a quick, nearly scarless operation.

Who's a candidate for this procedure? Anyone who thinks bigger would be better. Despite what you may have read in women's magazines and advertisements about herbal creams that are supposed to make your breasts grow (wouldn't *that* be nice?) or those new miracle "suction" bras that purportedly stimulate new breast tissue growth, implants are the only way you'll get significant and lasting results. Remember, though, that implants have mass—often up to two pounds each—and are relatively firm to the touch. So if you're bothered by the idea of toting around foreign objects in your body, implants probably aren't for you. On the health front, if you have a history of fibrocystic disease or dense breasts that complicate mammogram readings, implants may further aggravate these conditions. Confer with your plastic surgeon and primary care physician before undergoing surgery.

The Safety Issue

The questions I'm asked most from prospective patients are, *Are implants safe? Will they give me some sort of immune disorder? Can they cause cancer?* Many people remember the silicone implant scare of the early 1990s, when the FDA withdrew from the market silicone for use in implants because its leakage seemed linked to all sorts of complications, from inflammation to autoimmune diseases such as arthritis or chronic fatigue syndrome. When silicone implants were developed, the primary concern wasn't safety, but authenticity—developing implants that looked and felt like the real thing, and you can't beat silicone for that. But we've since learned that liquid silicone can cause local inflammation when it comes in contact with body tissue. The connection to autoimmune disease, however, was never proven, partly because women are much more prone to such disorders than men are. Although the FDA is currently conducting a controlled study to reevaluate silicone's viability in implants, we avoid using it except in breast reconstruction following mastectomy, when it is desirable because it offers the most natural appearance, and the silicone cannot leach into breast tissue if none is present.

Today's implants are very safe. They're filled with saline, or sterile salt water, the same fluid you use to clean your contact lenses. If an implant ruptures, there are no health consequences, because the body harmlessly absorbs the saline.

Breast health was of paramount concern to Gabrielle, a twenty-seven-year-old mother of twins whose sister Micki had recently been treated for breast cancer. Gabrielle had always been an A cup, but her pregnancy had left her breasts flat as pancakes, and she wanted to go to a C cup and eliminate some of the sag. She struggled with the decision to have implants, not only because she had trouble justifying to herself having a cosmetic procedure when Micki had just had a mastectomy, but also because she worried that she was somehow putting herself at increased risk for the disease. I reviewed with her some of the latest medical findings on the health effects of implants and assured her that there is no evidence that a breast implant increases your risk of getting a breast tumor. She finally came to see that putting her own life on hold wouldn't help her sister improve; in fact, having the surgery might have made her better able to help her sister when Micki got cosmetic breast reconstruction after her operation.

Another word about safety: Saline implants are encased in a silicone shell. Do you need to worry? Probably not. This kind of silicone can't get into your tissues. The only exception may be "textured" saline implants, which many doctors, including myself, started using a few years ago because they were thought to adhere better to the tissues and to reduce a common complication called capsular contracture, the formation of scar tissue around the implants. In the early 1990s, I was on a team that published a study showing that textured implants had the tendency to shed fragments of silicone into the surrounding tissue. On occasion, I still use these implants if someone is especially prone to capsulation (my personal feeling is that avoiding excessive scarring is worth the *very* remote risk of an implant fragmenting). But no safety issues have yet been associated with the smooth implants that are most commonly used. As for the cancer connection, a recent National Institutes of Health report that tracked breast-cancer rates in 13,500 women with both silicone and saline implants found that implant patients showed no increased risk for breast cancer.

New and *Not* Improved

You may have heard of other implant fillers that are available abroad or on the black market, including soybean and vegetable oils. Neither of these is

FDA-approved, and for good reason: Studies have shown that these substances trigger swelling and inflammation. Scientists are always experimenting with new implant technologies—currently under FDA review is a viscous silicone gel, which is less likely to leak than its predecessors, and hyaluronic acid, harvested from rooster combs. It's probable that new fillers will eventually be available.

The Right Fit

Just as clothing styles change with the seasons, so do breast implant preferences: large or small, round or perky. Over the years, there has been a steady stream of new implant models of different widths and shapes. A recent introduction is the "anatomical," or teardrop-shaped implant, which looks so authentic that no one will suspect you don't have the real thing. These are tricky to insert and require more precise placement, so many surgeons don't even offer them to patients.

Still, there are plenty of women who care less about looking natural than they do about having the kind of pop-up effect you get with a Wonderbra, and who am I to question their taste? In fact, 90 percent of the implants I used to do were anatomically shaped; then, in the last couple of years, a parade of women have come to me seeking the fuller, "Demi Moore" look. For them, I recommend a round implant: breasts that somewhat resemble half-grapefruits. They're very popular since they can be inserted easily through a tiny incision under the breast or nipple, or even through the armpit or navel.

Once you decide on a shape, how do you know what size is right for you? Most women want to get to an average size, a large B cup or a C cup. Typically, a patient and I will opt for a minimum size of 200 cubic centimeters (ccs) (the equivalent of 200 milliliters, or a little less than one liquid cup), but I have many patients who want to go larger than that.

Take Gabrielle, the patient whose sister had breast cancer. Like many flat-chested women who hate the way clothes fit them, she regularly wore silicone inserts or "cutlets" in her bra. "I'd just grown used to them over the years," she says. Then, suddenly, she got a taste of the real thing. "When I had children, I saw my body change drastically," she recalls. "Although I didn't nurse my babies, after I gave birth my breasts got so big from the milk coming in, I thought, 'If this is what I'd look like with implants, I'm doing it!' It's not like I wanted to come out looking like Pamela Anderson. But I really felt like I looked like a boy no matter how feminine my clothes. It frustrated me that there was this one aspect I could never change about my appearance despite all the hours I spent in the gym trying to look better."

I had proposed a B-plus cup in keeping with Gabrielle's rather slight build. But she wanted to recapture what she'd seen in the mirror, and so we went up to a C. It looked good; the size was still within reason for her height and weight. (I tell patients who insist on super-sizing their breasts that doing so can result in back and neck pain and other complications; when I feel a size is totally inadvisable, I won't perform the operation.) Gabrielle recalls the result: "I just felt more womanly and attractive. I could finally wear shirts and dresses that were low in the back, which was impossible with silicone inserts. I don't even need a bra when I'm at home because they barely sag at all. So in a way, they're better than the real thing!" (While it may be fun, I don't advise going without support if you don't have to—it's a surefire way to promote sagging.)

Just discussing size with your doctor isn't enough. I learned that the hard way years ago when I was starting out as a plastic surgeon. A patient wanted to go bigger, and we talked at length about what I was going to do. At the end of the operation, I stepped back to evaluate my work: Her breasts looked fabulous. My nurse and anesthesiologist agreed. Usually I require my patients to wear a special supportive bra and cotton dressing for a week after surgery, but this woman was so eager to take a peek after one day, I let her. When she caught a glimpse of her breasts, she got horribly upset; they were smaller than she wanted. It turns out there was a particular bra she'd hoped to be able to fill out after her procedure, but she'd never communicated that to me.

The experience taught me a valuable lesson. Now I tell all my implant patients to shop for a bra that they want to be able to fill out when the surgery is over. To make sure it's the right size, I tell them to stuff it with socks, hose, or whatever, and to walk around like that for a day, spending plenty of time in front of a mirror. Then I have them bring in the bra, which I sterilize, and at the end of surgery we try it on. If they fill it out, then I've done my job. If the breasts bulge out of the top or sink down into it, then I make a small adjustment by removing or adding fluid.

Some people have asked me, Wouldn't it be nice if there were adjustable implants that let you add and remove liquid without more surgery? There are, but I don't recommend them. First, it's not as if you can adjust them ad nauseum, as if they're beach balls. Once the patient settles on a size, the tube is removed and the incision is sewn up for good. Second, and more important, because adjustable implants are subject to more manipulation than regular ones, there's a greater chance of infection. If you and your doctor have a good, open line of communication, you shouldn't need to go back and forth—or up and down—on your decision.

Age, height, and weight also help to determine what size implant to get. Round, perky breasts would look pretty silly on a seventy-year-old woman, just as D cups would be inappropriate for a tiny-framed woman. Not that I am (or should be) the last word on what your breasts should look like. The surgical process is collaborative, and I often put in implants bigger than I might have chosen for the patient—so long as I think it's safe—because that's what she thinks will make her happy; and according to a recent survey, nearly a quarter of augmentation patients think they should have gone even bigger. So I leave that choice to my patients.

Over or Under?

Another factor that affects how breast implants look and feel is whether they're inserted over or under the chest (pectoral) muscle. Traditionally we do a *submammary implant*, inserting the implants *under* the breast tissue and *over* the muscle, because it's technically a lot easier (displacing the chest muscle requires a little more delicacy). It's also quicker: We just insert the implant through an incision in the navel, nipple, breast fold, or armpit, place it over the muscle, and then inflate it when it's snugly in place. The result is fabulous: perkiness with barely a trace of scar.

If you want the most natural-looking breast, however, you'll need a *subpectoral implant*, in which the implant is placed *under* the muscle. This procedure also requires the merest incision—about three centimeters in the crease under the breast or at the edge of the nipple—and diminishes the incidence of capsular contracture, the formation of hard scar tissue around the implant, which occurs in 10 to 30 percent of cases.

Subpectoral implants aren't right for everyone, though. If you have saggy breasts, an implant placed under the muscle won't fill out that empty breast sack, and you'll get what we call the "double bubble" look, where the implant is situated next to your armpit and the breast hangs several inches below it. Instead, you can have a combination procedure called *augmentation mastopexy*, in which the implant is placed under the muscle and the skin on the breast is lifted and tightened.

In short, you must know—realistically—what you're starting with, as well as what you want to look like when the surgery is done. Do you care more about the placement of the scar or about a quick, painless procedure? Do you want a natural appearance or a round, perky look? These are some of the factors I weigh with my patients when evaluating what type of procedure to do.

GETTING READY FOR BREAST SURGERY

As with any procedure, you should avoid spicy and salty foods and alcohol (which promote inflammation) the day before surgery; steer clear of aspirin and anti-inflammatory medications for *two weeks prior*. Read your doctor's pre-op instructions carefully, and consult Chapter 12 in this book for more details.

What the Surgery Involves

Breast augmentation is routinely performed in a surgeon's office. You will likely be given a local anesthetic and twilight sedation for one to two hours, so you'll be relaxed but won't feel groggy during recovery. There are four common types of incisions, each about an inch and a half long:

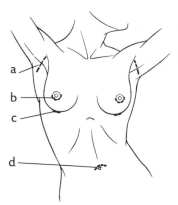

COMMON INCISIONS
FOR BREAST
AUGMENTATION

◆ **Axillary incision (a).** A tiny incision is made in the armpit; remarkably, the surgeon snakes the implant through there using either a hollow tube or an endoscope, so that the implant lies either over or under the muscle.

◆ **Periareolar incision (b).** Made on the edge of the areola just below the nipple, this incision is the most concealed, as it can blend into the surrounding areolar color.

◆ **Inframammary incision (c).** The most common type, this incision is made in the crease below the breast, and is well hidden in the skin's natural fold.

◆ **Umbilical incision (d).** Discreetly concealed in the navel, this incision is an option only for those getting round implants, which are snaked into place under the skin using an endoscope. It would be too difficult to position an anatomical implant starting all the way down at the navel.

Once the incision is made, the surgeon creates a pocket into which the implant is inserted. This pocket is located either directly behind the breast tissue (submammary) or beneath the pectoral muscle underlying the breast tissue (subpectoral). Afterward, the implants are filled with salt water. To minimize scarring, your surgeon may suture the incisions on the underside of the skin.

Recovery

When you wake up, you'll probably feel as if your breasts are pushed up to your chin. Part of this is imaginary. As to the part that's real, don't panic: The swelling goes down in about two weeks. If you have a subpectoral implant, you'll likely feel some pain, because the muscle has been stretched to accommodate the implant. Most patients of mine who've had submammary implants, on the

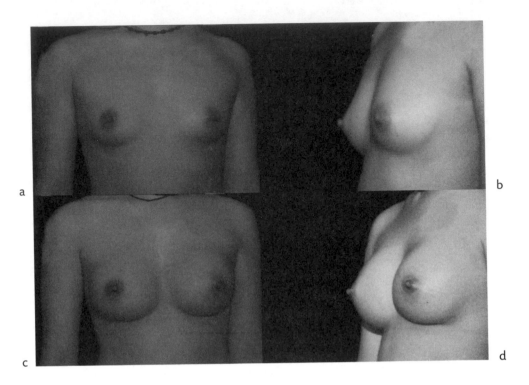

a

b

c

d

BREAST AUGMENTATION WITH ANATOMICALLY SHAPED IMPLANTS

This eighteen-year-old college athlete was a 34A when she came to see me about breast augmentation (a, b). In keeping with her slight build (5'5", 115 pounds), she wanted to increase to a B cup to maintain a natural look. I told her we could achieve that goal using "anatomically shaped" implants (in her case, 330 cubic centimeters of saline) placed under the pectoral muscle. She didn't want any scars to be visible, so we hid them discreetly in the inframammary fold beneath her breasts (c, d).

other hand, report little or no discomfort. "When I woke up, the nurse was putting my shirt on," recalls Chantal, the twenty-seven-year-old actress who went from an A cup to a C. "It was a struggle to lift my arms—they felt as if they were stuck to my sides—but I didn't feel any pain whatsoever."

Since surgeons never agree on anything, post-op routines vary. Some doctors tape the breasts down to keep them in place while they heal; others put a strap across the chest. Either way, for at least one week you will be required to

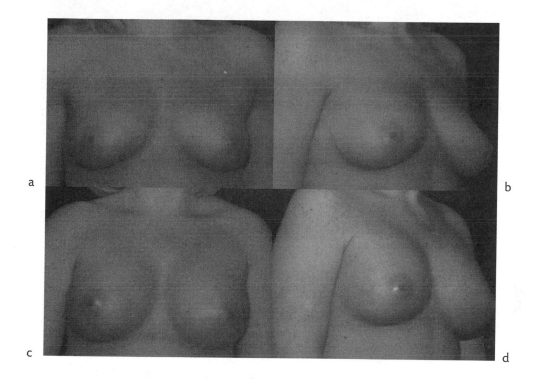

a
b
c
d

BREAST AUGMENTATION WITH ROUND IMPLANTS

A not-so-flat 34B, this 5'3", sales rep in her thirties wanted to go bigger—and better (a, b). She yearned for cleavage, which meant getting fuller on top, the kind of look one can get only from a "round" implant. Through incisions in the breasts' inframammary folds, I inserted implants under the pectoral muscles and filled them with 360 cubic centimeters of saline. By putting the implants under the muscles, I was able to keep the breasts from sagging (c, d). Today she is a D cup, and extremely happy with her appearance.

wear a very supportive bra—we have a special surgical one that buttons in the front—and a soft cotton dressing. This makes showering tough, but you may find the bra so snug and comforting that you won't want to take it off at the end of the week. Remember to wear comfortable clothing you can easily slip into after the operation—in other words, nothing that requires you to lift your arms over your head!

Breast implants usually don't complicate mammogram readings, but they may. I've seen implants rupture as a result of the mammogram, especially when the implant is situated under the breast tissue and not the muscle wall. Also, the place in the breast where the implant and tissue meet can be difficult to read. Be sure to find a radiologist experienced in imaging breasts with implants, one who has specialized equipment that's able to take extra views to get the most accurate reading.

Common Side Effects

Moderate Pain, Constriction, and "Unwieldiness"

Swelling may cause you to feel uncomfortable pressure and soreness for a week or so; you may also feel as if you're wearing bowling balls. This hardness and heaviness subsides within six weeks to three months. Generally, though, if you experience more than moderate pain, call your doctor.

Blood and Fluid Leakage

This may continue for up to four days after the operation. For the first twenty-four hours, you may be required to wear drains at the incision sites—rubber tubes connected to a reservoir that collect any blood or liquid that may seep out.

Bruising

You're most likely to be black and blue either under the breasts or arms, depending on where your incisions are. These symptoms may continue for up to three weeks, though some patients have almost no bruising whatsoever.

Nipple Numbness

If you had a periareolar incision, you may experience decreased sensation around the nipple. With the other types of incisions, no loss of sensation should occur.

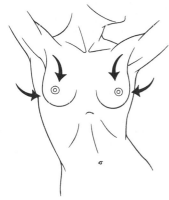

BREAST
MANIPULATION
EXERCISE

Scar Irritation

Scars are a fact (and artifact) of surgery. At first, they will appear red and lumpy; after four to six weeks they will be smoother and less fiery. To help reduce a scar's vividness, your doctor may give you a steroid cream, silicone gel, or pigment blocker. Do not try to treat the scars yourself with homeopathic remedies without consulting your surgeon.

The bottom line is that just one day after surgery, you'll be up and around. You can go to a movie, for a walk, even to work, so long as you're not doing anything strenuous or that would make you sweat and interrupt the healing process. At the end of the first week, I change the dressing and require my patients to have a lymphatic massage, a light-touch technique that helps the body heal by mobilizing the lymphatic fluids that contribute to swelling (for more on massage technique, see Chapter 12). Since scar tissue in the breasts tends to contract from the top and sides, I have patients do five minutes of light exercises, see illustration—pushing the breasts in from the sides and down from the top—a few times a day for several weeks.

Side Effects to Be Concerned About

Capsular Contracture

The formation of tough scar tissue around the implant—the body's way of protecting itself from a foreign object—occurs in 10 to 30 percent of patients, and is experienced as a painful hardening of the breast. (In extreme and rare cases, capsular contracture results in a displacement of the implant, necessitating repeat surgery.) You can help to avoid this by gently manipulating your breasts in and down.

Deflation/Rupture

About 5 percent of implants leak, deflate immediately, or deflate gradually over several days. This is typically caused by intense manipulation or compression. If the implant is leaky, it must be replaced. Fortunately, the body simply absorbs the sterile saline and there is no health risk.

Loss of Nipple Sensation

In rare cases, the numbness experienced in the first weeks after surgery can be permanent, especially in the case of a periareolar incision, where nerves in the area may have been severed.

Hematoma

A hematoma is a pooling of blood under the skin in the days following surgery that may be caused by excessive internal bleeding, physical activity, or high blood pressure. Risk is extremely small (about 2 percent), though it is higher among those who take aspirin or ibuprofen or who resume vigorous activity too soon after surgery.

Infection

As with any surgery, there's always a chance of infection. To minimize the risk, you may be put on a preventive cycle of antibiotics for one week.

URGENT QUESTION:

WILL I BE ABLE TO BREASTFEED AFTER GETTING IMPLANTS?

Many implant patients worry about how childbirth will affect their breasts. During pregnancy, your breasts should enlarge normally, with no consequence to the implants. Implants shouldn't affect the ability to breastfeed, especially if they're placed under the chest muscle wall. It *is* possible that you'll feel some pain when your breasts become engorged (most nursing mothers do, anyway), because your skin has already been stretched to the max. If you plan to have children after getting implants, talk to your doctor about it.

Adjusting to New Breasts

My patients tend to be ecstatic when they first see their new, fuller breasts. "I wanted to jump up and down, which of course would have hurt terribly!" recalls Gabrielle. "I just wanted to go outside and show them off," says Chantal. At the outset, your breasts may feel very full on top, quite firm, and also very high, as if you're channeling Dolly Parton. As the swelling goes down over the next three months, they will feel softer and smaller.

Still, it may take some time to adjust to your new size. After all, the weight of your breasts may have a noticeable effect on your posture and gait. "It was a bit of an identity crisis," admits Gabrielle. You will immediately notice that you wear your clothes differently (those waistless dresses and loose-fitting shirts will now tend to make you look boxy), but it can be exciting to shop for form-fitting clothes, halter tops, and bras.

Prepare yourself to feel as if your breasts are on public display, because they are. Many women report feeling ogled—at work, at social gatherings, and on the street. While it may not be the kind of attention you were initially seeking, many women enjoy its novelty. "I notice guys looking at my breasts all the time, especially at the gym, since for the first time in my life I'm exercising in a sports bra and feel really comfortable with it," says Chantal. "I don't mind the stares—part of me feels like that was the point!"

Yours for Life?

Manufacturers claim that breast implants will last seven to ten years before the risk of rupture increases (silicone wears when it rubs), but that doesn't mean

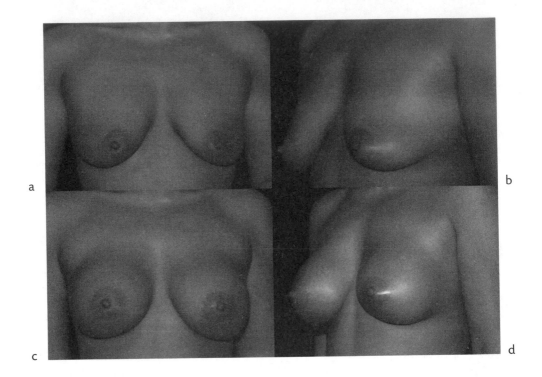

a

b

c

d

LIFT THROUGH BREAST AUGMENTATION

When women with saggy breasts want to go bigger, I usually advise doing a breast lift along with the implants. Otherwise, the implants create what we call a "double bubble," where the breast droops off the end of the implant like a sock. This thirty-five-year-old attorney didn't want a lift, though, because she hoped to avoid additional scarring. So I arrived at another solution: "round" implants, which create greater fullness on top. I placed these under the breast tissue and filled them with 230 cubic centimeters of saline—quite a lot for a petite woman of 5'1"—in order to fill out the skin. In the end, she became a 34C and didn't look saggy at all.

you'll be due for an upgrade at that point. Patients of mine have worn the same implants for twenty years with no problem. And at the conclusion of your surgery, you should receive a manufacturer's warranty for replacement in the event of rupture.

A NOTE ABOUT BREAST RECONSTRUCTION

Today, treatment of breast cancer no longer entails extensive operations that leave patients mutilated and disfigured. Thanks to early detection and advances in reconstructive techniques, the breast can continue to look and feel quite real. One patient, who had breast reconstruction surgery after a radical mastectomy, even said that her new boyfriend didn't realize until her clothes were off that her breast wasn't "real."

The breast reconstruction method you opt for depends on your medical situation, breast shape and size, and body type. We can reconstruct the breast by using a prosthesis (either a silicone gel or saline-filled breast implant), your own tissues (a "tissue flap"), or a combination of the two. A tissue flap is a section of skin, fat, and muscle that is relocated from your stomach or back to the chest area and shaped into a breast. The nipple is usually reconstructed using a skin graft from the chest area. The procedure is often performed at the same time as the mastectomy, but it can also be done months or even years after a patient has had a mastectomy or a reconstruction whose appearance she wants to improve.

BREAST LIFT (MASTOPEXY)

The body is subject to the laws of gravity, and breasts are Exhibit A. As we age, breast tissue loses elasticity and fat, and droops or sags. Other factors make breasts go south, too. Mothers may find that pregnancy and breastfeeding contribute to loss of volume and firmness, while women who've lost a lot of weight tend to have saggy breasts because the skin has been stretched. Women who in their youth proudly paraded around braless are now paying for that esprit de corps.

Implants aren't the only way to restore youthfulness to breasts: Another popular option is the breast lift (*mastopexy*), in which droopy breasts are raised from one to several inches and excess skin is removed.

How do you know if you're a candidate for implants or a lift? First, ask yourself whether your problem is volume or shape. If you want to go bigger,

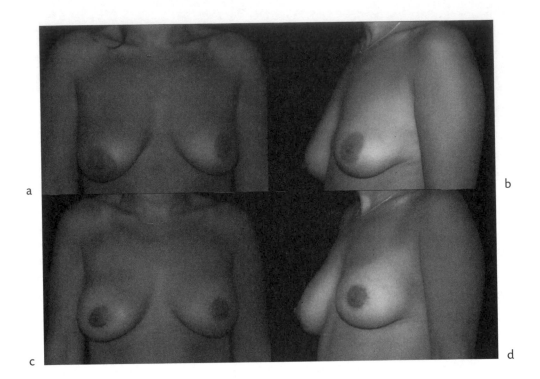

a

b

c

d

AUGMENTATION MASTOPEXY

Sometimes, one breast is larger or saggier than the other (a). This thirty-four-year-old woman, a 34B, didn't like the asymmetry of her breasts and wanted more fullness on top (b). Because her breasts were *both* somewhat saggy, however, an implant alone wouldn't have sufficed: She also needed a lift. I performed both—the lift and the implant insertion—through a periareolar incision, running around the nipple. The lift allowed putting the implants underneath the pectoral muscle. To even out the size of the breasts I added five or ten extra cubic centimeters of saline to the left implant. Now the woman's breasts are far more symmetrical and fuller, and she is much happier (c, d).

the only way to get that result is with implants. If you're sagging or asymmetrical and are looking for perkiness, you'll need a lift—or, if you also want more volume, a lift *and* implants. And by the way, droop isn't subjective: Horrifying as it sounds, doctors actually have precise anatomical measurements for defining pendulousness (the clinical term is *ptosis*). Basically, if your nipple hangs below the breast fold, then you've got sag.

What the Surgery Involves

To perk up a drooping breast, your surgeon will remove excess skin, reposition the nipple, and redrape and tighten the remaining skin to support the breast. The areola may be reduced in size. The whole procedure takes between two and three hours and is performed using a local anesthetic with twilight sedation (my preference), or general anesthesia.

There are three main lift techniques, each targeting a specific problem and requiring a different set of incisions. Each technique also yields a slightly different look, so ask your surgeon to show you the range of results:

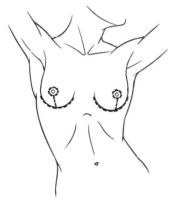

**INFERIOR PEDICLE
INCISIONS**

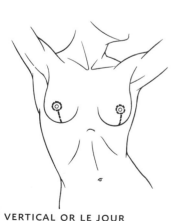

**VERTICAL OR LE JOUR
INCISIONS**

◆ **The inferior pedicle technique** (see illustration). Though I hardly use it anymore, this procedure is still the standard option for many surgeons, typically used to correct pronounced droop. However, it also leaves the most scarring. An incision is made around the areola, another runs vertically down to the breast fold, and a third is made in the crease underneath the breast, also known as the inframammary fold (your scar will look like an inverted T, or sometimes a J or L). The surgeon removes excess breast skin, creating a pedicle, or tissue base, that is used to carry the nipple and areola to a higher position. Skin that was formerly above the areola is brought down and joined beneath it, to reshape the breast.

How much the nipple is repositioned varies from patient to patient. Most surgeons no longer completely detach the nipple, as was once done. Instead, the nipple is left attached to the underlying tissue, milk ducts, and nerve endings, and just sewn into a higher position. That way, breastfeeding and nipple sensation should remain unaffected by surgery.

◆ **The vertical or Le Jour technique** (see illustration). This technique was pioneered for smaller-breasted women and those with moderate droop, but can now

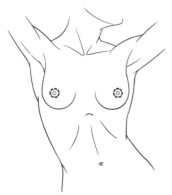

PERIAREOLAR OR
"PURSESTRING"
INCISIONS

be used on a wide range of sizes. It results in a perky, conical breast that many women find desirable. The resulting incision from this procedure looks like a lollipop: The same cut is made around the areola as with the inferior pedicle, but it connects to a vertical incision down the lower half of the breast.

◆ **The periareolar or "pursestring" technique** (see illustration). This is best for women whose breasts aren't overly droopy. It results in virtually no visible scarring and a rounded shape. With an incision around the areola, the skin is pulled together with a "gather" stitch, just like in sewing. The only downside of the periareolar method is that it leaves a kind of puckered appearance, but this smooths out after a few months.

Recovery

Your breasts will be bruised and swollen for one to two weeks. You will have to wear a surgical bra with cotton dressings for about a week, which is then replaced by a soft, supportive bra of your choice that must be worn for a month, even when you sleep. Recovery takes a little longer than it does after implant surgery because there are more (and longer) incisions. You probably won't feel like returning to work for at least three days. Lifting heavy weights and doing any exercise that will cause you to sweat, which can bring bacteria to the area and increase the risk of infection, are forbidden for about two weeks. After several weeks, you can build back to a regular workout routine.

Common Side Effects

Soreness, Bruising, and Swelling
These symptoms may last for up to two weeks. To help prevent swelling, you may be given steroids before surgery; afterward, anti-inflammatories effectively combat the problem.

Nipple Numbness

This is almost always temporary; full feeling should return in six months to a year.

Scar Irritation

At first, incisions appear red and lumpy; after four to six weeks they are smoother and less fiery. To help reduce the scars' vividness and soften their texture, your doctor may give you a steroid cream, silicone gel, or pigment blocker.

Side Effects to Be Concerned About

As with any surgery, there is a small risk of post-operative infection, bleeding, or blood clots (hematomas). Other complications are similar to those described in the previous breast augmentation section (pages 157–158), with a few differences:

Noticeable Asymmetry

There may be minor variations between the two breasts; occasionally, the differences are more than minor. If so, the problem can be corrected with another procedure.

Nipple Complications

Permanent loss of nipple sensation, nipple inversion, or change of nipple color may occur.

"Bottoming Out"

Breast tissue, which can be quite heavy, may descend below the newly positioned nipple. This problem can be minimized, however, if the surgeon positions the nipple slightly lower on the breast than where you ultimately want it.

Keloid Scarring

Five to 10 percent of patients have scars that hypertrophy, or have excessive scar production. Of those, a fraction end up with permanent red, raised scars, or, in dark-skinned women, scars that are darker than the surrounding skin. The pigment and texture of the scar can be improved with steroid creams and injections, laser treatment, microdermabrasion, and pigment-blocking creams.

BREAST REDUCTION (MAMMOPLASTY)

Imagine walking around wearing a knapsack stuffed with five- to seven-pound sandbags—*all the time.* That's pretty much what it's like to have very large breasts—only you're wearing the knapsack in front, which is even harder for the body to support.

As any D-plus-cup woman knows, finding bras and clothes that fit can be a real challenge. Wearing a bathing suit or a form-fitting tank top is almost entirely out of the question. Unfortunately, because breasts are literally so front and center, when you have huge breasts your sense of physical self is that you're huge, even if the rest of you—torso, arms, and legs—is thin.

"My breasts always gave me a matronly look," says Laurie, who came to see me for a breast reduction—at age sixty-two. She had waited her whole life to do something about her large chest; even her obstetrician had urged her to have the procedure after the birth of her third child caused her breasts to inflate far beyond her regular D cup. At the time, however, she didn't have the money or the resolve. Years later, in her fifties, when another plastic surgeon—a man—performed a face-lift on her, she thought of having her breasts done at the same time, but "I was too embarrassed to get undressed in front of a male doctor," she recalls. "For all those years, I was humiliated even to get a mammogram. My breasts would just lie there on the machine looking so enormous—I don't even know how they were able to get a proper reading!" Now in her mid-sixties, Laurie's B-cup breasts give her greater confidence and ease of movement.

Large breasts can also literally restrict your lifestyle. Jogging, hiking, and other forms of exercise are a whole lot tougher when you're carrying around that kind of baggage, thus making weight control a hopeless battle. Even the performance of certain occupations is affected: Once, a patient of mine who was a seamstress said she couldn't get close enough to her table to work effectively because her breasts were so big.

More seriously, large breasts can cause a variety of medical problems, including back, neck, and shoulder pain; shoulder grooving from bra straps; bad posture and curvature of the spine; and chronic rashes under the breasts.

Ample endowment can be especially difficult for girls. Listen to Eliza, a nineteen-year-old college student I operated on:

"I have always been overweight, and since puberty I've had large breasts—36D. In high school I played field hockey and lacrosse, and wore two sports bras at once. Even so, I was slower than everyone, and my breasts hurt when I ran. I had gouges in my shoulders from my bra straps, and my back always hurt. My mom told me that if I lost weight my breasts would go down. Well, I lost fifty pounds and they didn't change at all. At that point, she told me I'd earned having surgery."

I explained to Eliza that her weight had very little to do with the size of her breasts. She was excited and relieved to hear that we could do something about her problem. She continues:

"After the operation, the second I stood up I felt different . . . much lighter. The whole thing has made a major change in my life—everything is so much easier and not at all painful. I work out every day, and I can run farther and faster than I used to. I can even wear button-down shirts and tank tops and normal bras. I have a lot more self-confidence, and that comes out when I'm around other people."

In short, she can live the life a nineteen-year-old girl is entitled to.

ARE YOU OLD ENOUGH FOR BREAST REDUCTION?

During puberty, the mammary glands in the breasts respond to hormonal changes by enlarging. While breasts may continue to grow into a woman's early twenties, most women are fully developed by age sixteen. If a teenager is a DD cup, she's certainly not going to get any smaller. So if the size of her breasts is debilitating or painful, I would suggest going ahead with a reduction. She may need a second reductive procedure down the line, but why put off something that could make such a positive difference in her life now?

Overweight and Overcharged

Many patients who were considered clinically obese have come to me despondent, after being turned away by other surgeons who refused to perform breast reduction surgery on them until they lost weight. I find taking that position ridiculous. Although breasts are comprised partly of fat, even drastic weight loss won't result in more than negligible shrinkage in that area (and even then, the breasts will still be saggy). Many doctors ignore a crucial dilemma: When your breasts are so large, exercise is a miserable, if not impossible, option. How exactly are you supposed to drop pounds?

Being overweight doesn't exclude you from having breast reduction surgery. In fact, it will motivate you to lose weight by improving your body image and freeing you to exercise with minimal bouncing and flopping.

What the Surgery Involves

In breast reduction, your surgeon not only reduces the size of the breasts by removing excess tissue and fat, but sculpts them into a new, smaller shape. I always do the procedure under local anesthesia and twilight sedation, though some doctors still use a general anesthetic. Expect to be in the operating room for three to four hours.

The most common techniques are the same as those outlined in the breast lift section (see illustrations on pages 163 and 164). Basically, tissue and fat are

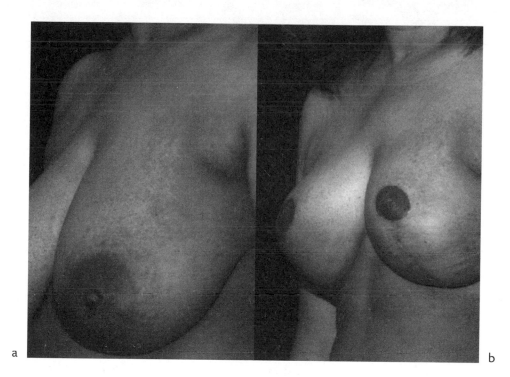

a   b

LE JOUR BREAST REDUCTION

This fifty-two-year-old nurse was a 36DDD(a)—so large, in fact, that she had trouble even going about her work! Black skin tends to show scars more prominently than white skin, so I opted to use the Le Jour (or vertical) reduction technique, where the incision runs just around the nipple and down to the fold in the breast (b). After becoming a C cup, she embarked on an exercise program for the first time in her life and lost fifteen pounds, further improving her body's proportions.

---

taken from the bottom of your breast and your nipple and areola are relocated to a higher position. Since big-breasted women tend to have very large nipples, we usually reduce the size of the areola, too. By leaving intact the stem of the nipple—the part that connects to the milk ducts—we minimize the risk that you will lose nipple sensation or function. In the case of gigantomastia, where the breasts are extremely large or pendulous, some doctors may use a "free-nipple graft," in which the nipple is detached, because of the consider-

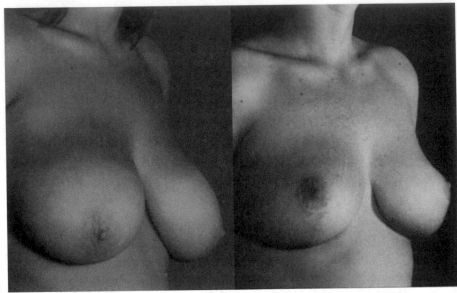

a   b

BREAST REDUCTION USING INFERIOR PEDICLE METHOD

The traditional breast reduction incision, called an inferior pedicle, is something I rarely do anymore since newer techniques (the Le Jour and periareolar methods) leave a less prominent scar. But many doctors still favor this method, in which the incision runs around the nipple, down to the inframammary fold, and then horizontally underneath the fold. This eighteen-year-old high school student worried that her D-cup chest looked like "an old lady's bosom (a)." The inferior pedicle created the perky-looking breasts she wanted (b).

---

able distance that the nipple has to be raised. But this technique isn't always necessary, so if your doctor is recommending it, seek a second opinion.

Some women fear ending up with different sized breasts. Your surgeon knows exactly how much tissue he or she is taking out, because it is weighed after removal. And breast reduction comes with an added bonus: The extracted breast tissue is always sent to a lab and examined by a pathologist for signs of cysts or cancer.

Recovery

When you wake up after a breast reduction, you'll probably feel some pain, especially if you cough. Recovery is roughly the same as after mastopexy—you'll have to wear a surgical bra for a week, and then a supportive bra for four to six weeks, day and night. You should avoid any jarring exercise for at least one month. But there are a few differences between reduction and a lift:

◆ Since reduction is more invasive than just a lift, there will likely be more bleeding on the first day. Your surgeon may insert drains to siphon off any excess fluid.

◆ Although you'll have an idea of how your new breasts will look within three weeks or so, they won't take on their ultimate shape for several months.

◆ Tissue dissection will likely result in a few days or weeks of breast tenderness. You'll want to wait six months before having your routine mammogram, just to be sure the healing is complete.

"My recovery really wasn't painful, though I was quite sore for a few days," recalls Laurie, on whom I used a vertical, or Le Jour, incision to go from a D cup to a B. "The worst part was that for two days you wear drains, and there's all sorts of gross stuff that comes out. You have to be motivated to get through it. I took off two whole weeks from work, but I played golf after three weeks, so I probably could have gone back to the office sooner."

Light as a Feather

"I'm free!" You might just find yourself cheering your own liberation when you stand up and feel your new lightness. You'll also see how smaller breasts can take years—and pounds—off of your appearance. Go home and toss out all those big, drapey shirts and sweaters that used to give you "mono-breast." You'll look terrific in fitted clothes that flatter your new form. And then get yourself over to Victoria's Secret and treat yourself to a cute bra that doesn't have a double letter in the size.

"For the first time in my life," says Laurie, "clothes shopping is fun. If I like something, I can buy it. I just picked out a 'normal' bathing suit, one that doesn't have 'bones' inside of it. I can fit into the bras I wore before I had kids—many of which I kept!—and they're so comfortable. Life in general is so much easier. I'm kicking myself that I didn't have the surgery earlier."

URGENT QUESTION: *WILL I BE ABLE TO BREASTFEED AFTER REDUCTION SURGERY?*

Though there is no guarantee, plenty of women are able to breastfeed successfully after breast reduction. Since milk ducts and nipples are usually left intact, lactation is unlikely to be affected by surgery. In fact, because nursing with extremely large breasts can be uncomfortable, if not physically impossible, many women who undergo reduction surgery opt to breastfeed post-surgery who wouldn't have done so before. If you're planning on becoming pregnant at some point, ask your doctor to explain the risks in more detail.

Liposuction: A New Way to Reduce

Recently, I and other surgeons started using liposuction for breast reduction. This technique delivers super results, though it isn't right for everyone. If you have good skin quality and minimal sagging, you make an ideal candidate for reduction using lipo alone. (Sometimes I use lipo in conjunction with one of the other breast reduction techniques.) Lipo is also a quick and effective way of correcting breast asymmetry.

How does it work? We just make a tiny incision of a few millimeters underneath the breast and with a cannula suck out some of the fat and tissue. Since lipo stimulates the skin to tighten around the affected area, the breasts actually lift a little bit. The procedure takes about an hour, the recovery takes just a couple of days, and there's virtually no scarring. This is such a fabulous option that I have even used it on older women patients who want to lose volume, but don't care about sagging. For young patients with large breasts, a lipo reduction may prevent breast sag from ever occurring!

URGENT QUESTION: *WHO PICKS UP THE TAB?*

Breast reduction is usually covered by insurance when the surgery is performed as part of a medically mandated procedure to treat neck, back, or shoulder pain or other problems related to the spine. Recently, managed care has adopted stricter standards for coverage, so these problems have to be thoroughly documented in writing by your primary care physician and plastic surgeon. They may also have to submit photographs. Even then, you may be required to seek a second opinion from a chiropractor, physical therapist, or orthopedic surgeon. Your best bet is to find a plastic surgeon who is willing to be your advocate and deal personally with the health insurance organization.

In short, breasts are one of the easiest parts of the body to change, since the incisions we use for implants, lifts, and reductions are smaller than ever, the healing time is short, and you can conceal your surgery under clothing and thus return sooner to your public life. In the following chapter, we'll look at the latest and best ways to recontour the *entire* body, neck to ankle.

10

The Body: Recontouring Through Liposuction, Lifts, and Tucks

I can do more for overweight people in one afternoon than they can do for themselves in a year. I have patients who have gone, literally overnight, from a size 12 to a size 8.

Both women and men are constantly at war with certain cursed parts of their bodies whose imperfections and excess fat have everything to do with DNA or hormones, and not with some innate lack of character. Dimply thighs, bulging tummy, "riding britches" on a woman's hips, love handles around a man's waist, elephant ankles—if one of these trouble zones is in your genetic cards, then all your good intentions and hours on the treadmill and desserts not ordered won't help. "Spot reduction," as it's optimistically called, doesn't work, either. Your deposit of fat cells, the one you've been pinching and obsessing over for years, is as much a heritable predisposition as your eye color and hair texture.

Body recontouring—the surgical removal of fat and skin and the molding of muscle—is something we plastic surgeons have long been doing in one form or another. Until recently, however, even the most popular recontouring procedures left patients with obtrusive scars, rippled skin, and otherwise mediocre results. Today, liposuction and new lifting and tucking techniques make it possible to transform a body's shape with less visible, or even no, scarring.

The recontouring revolution has transformed the lives of millions of men and women. I know that sounds like an exaggeration, but imagine what it's like for a woman who for decades concealed her thighs under A-line skirts to now wear shorts, unselfconsciously, on a hot summer day. Or for a man who has shed 150 pounds through dieting and exercise to have layers of excess skin (and the accompanying stretch marks) excised, leaving him with a boyishly flat back and abdomen. Or for a young mother whose stomach never snapped back following the birth of twins to be able to wear a bikini again.

The body is a work in progress. Although there's no substitute for good diet and exercise, sometimes there's only so much we can do to reverse nature's cruelties. That's where science comes in. No, reshaping your body isn't as easy as going to the beauty parlor: Surgery is never 100-percent risk-free, and for many procedures, especially those that require skin removal, the healing process requires patience and determination. My job, then, is to help you determine which procedure or procedures (for I will often use liposuction first, and resort to a lift only when necessary) will give you the results you want, and make you proud to show the world your arms or thighs or stomach or hips, perhaps for the first time in your adult life. Here, I discuss the differences among the newest recontouring techniques, and how to make an informed choice about what's right for you.

LIPOSUCTION: THE SKINNY

Liposuction modifies volume and contour, or "sculpts," by sucking out fat that collects disproportionately in certain areas. For a veteran dieter, it may be her "pinch-an-inch" love handles. For an otherwise conditioned workout zealot, it may be a butt that's unjustly big for her frame. For a man, it may be enlarged breasts or a double chin. There are countless such individuals and dissatisfying body parts. For them, lipo is a potential godsend.

Still, many people feel as if it's cheating to use liposuction to eliminate fat that's been irritating them forever. Such rapid reduction feels, well, *unearned*: a shortcut, a blow to our cherished "no pain, no gain" ethic.

Stop punishing yourself. You've tried your best; it didn't work. Now let's move on to Plan B.

Alyssa had been exercising vigorously for years, working out with trainers, taking aerobics classes and TaeBo. "Whatever new trend came out, I tried," recalls the twenty-five-year-old medical student. "But I could never reduce the size of my thighs or butt. I once heard that it's ideal to have a ten-inch difference between your waist and your hips, but I had a fifteen-inch difference! With those proportions, it just seemed like I wasn't going to get anywhere the natural way."

Alyssa had a little bit of money saved up from her former job in consulting, and came in to see me. Together, we used computer imaging to visualize the goal she wanted to reach. Eventually, I performed liposuction on Alyssa's buttocks and outer thighs. Her boyfriend, who had been skeptical at the outset, loved the results so much he bought her another round of lipo for Valentine's Day (a much more enduring gift than a dozen roses!). Recently, she returned to have her inner thighs, knees, and triceps done. "I still exercise every other day," says Alyssa, "but I get so much more out of it now that I can actually see the fruits of my training, instead of their being obscured by a layer of fat."

A Weighty Decision

Liposuction is by far the most popular procedure I perform, and the most requested type of cosmetic surgery in the United States. In the year 2001, more than 307,000 American women got lipoed. In one form or another, liposuction is employed in nearly three-quarters of all cosmetic procedures. A face-lift on a heavy person, for example, is usually more successful when the jowls and double chin are lipoed, too. Liposuction has unquestionably revolutionized my field.

For optimal results, lipo candidates need good skin tone. Younger skin has an obvious advantage: Because lipo stimulates skin to tighten and redrape, good elasticity provides a smooth contour after fat is removed. That's not to say that older people can't benefit from liposuction. I recently did back and abdomen lipos on a sixty-five-year-old, and she was thrilled to see improvements in areas that had bothered her for years. Her skin was obviously not as taut as a twenty-five- or forty-year-old's, but she looked markedly better. The real key to success? Her expectations were realistic.

Developed in France in the 1980s, traditional or suction-assisted liposuction employs a narrow, rigid, hollow tube called a cannula that is inserted in an incision near the problem area. To break up fat, the surgeon forcefully manipulates—jabs, really—the cannula, which is attached to a syringe or vacuum pump. As fat is broken up and siphoned, the area diminishes in size. This is where the surgeon's artistry comes in: Through feel and sight, he or she tries to make the fat-reduced area as smooth and symmetrical as possible. Once that's done, the incision is closed. That area will almost certainly never be a problem again.

How can that be? By the time we reach puberty, the number of fat cells in our system is set. Although each fat cell can fluctuate in size, getting smaller or larger depending on calorie intake and exercise, the actual number of cells doesn't change. Because of genetics, some areas simply house more fat cells than one wants. When we suction some of these cells from the problem area, we permanently reduce the amount of fat that can build up there. Some years ago, a study was done on animals in which their abdomens were suctioned, just the way it's done with humans, after which the animals were fed to obesity. They got fat, of course, but less fat was stored in the abdomen: The volume of fat cells simply wasn't there anymore to absorb the food.

THE FAT GENDER GAP

Any stroll down the beach reveals it: Men and women wear their fat differently. For women, extra weight tends to accumulate on the hips, thighs, and knees, whereas men carry their fat around their waist and abdomen. After menopause, a woman may find that she, too, gets thicker around the waist, thanks to a precipitous drop in female hormones like estrogen. There's even a difference in the quality and texture of our fat: A man's is firmer and more fibrous. As a result of these factors, surgeons use different instruments when performing lipo on men and women, and sculpt the body using disparate optimal proportions.

In the early days of liposuction, we practiced the technique differently. Then, the patient almost invariably required hospitalization, often for several days. The cannulas were larger and caused more trauma to the system; there was more blood loss; less fat could be removed; and irregularities in the skin such as dimpling and waviness were far more prevalent. Thanks to new technologies, these limitations are ancient history. By the 1990s, we were using narrower cannulas that enabled smaller incisions. Fat could be suctioned out at different angles and with greater precision, thus minimizing rippling on the treated area. Scars today are much smaller and more discreetly located. Also, a patient can undergo lipo without a sedative. Indeed, a long lunch hour may be all one needs to complete certain procedures.

Liposuction is not meant to solve a chronic weight problem, nor can it turn an obese person into a svelte one. It can help, certainly, but in extremely overweight people it can be dangerous and destabilizing to remove *too* much fat, too quickly. In fact, liposuction works best on patients who are of relatively average weight, but who need help with a problem area, or with shedding the ten pounds they regain between diets.

Take Diane, who came to me for liposuction six months after giving birth to her first child. At thirty-one, she didn't have a lifelong weight problem. "There was nothing wrong with me, per se, but having a baby is hard on the body and I wanted to get back to where I was before my pregnancy," she says. She had been exercising regularly since her son was six weeks old and hadn't seen much change in her shape. I liposuctioned her trouble spots: her arms, stomach, inner and outer thighs, and knees. I was able to do all these areas at once because I didn't remove too much fat from any one of them. For all of Diane's incision sites, she had only one healing period. Within three or four days just about all the swelling had gone down, and Diane was able to move around freely and pick up her baby without any discomfort.

Since the technology's inception, several types of liposuction have been developed. I use them all, often in combination, because each offers different advantages for certain body parts or types of fat. They are:

Traditional or Suction-Assisted Liposuction (SAL)

The granddaddy of lipo methods requires a forceful motion of the cannula to loosen and suck out fat. There may be significant (though not permanent) trauma to nerve and connective tissue, since in order to remove fat the cannula must break up the fibrous bands that connect the skin to muscle tissue. As a result, there is likely to be a good deal of bruising and swelling. If this method doesn't sound ideal, it isn't: Traditional lipo isn't employed as often as it once was except in the cheeks and face, where the cannulas we use are tiny and don't traumatize the surrounding areas.

Tumescent or "Super-Wet" Liposuction

Tumescent means "swollen." In this popular method, which I use in conjunction with almost every lipo procedure, a solution that contains epinephrine (adrenaline) and an anesthetic (usually lidocaine) is injected into the area to be treated. This constricts blood vessels while also bloating fat pockets, making it easier to manipulate the cannula under the skin. There is less jabbing and more continuous movement. Underlying muscle and tissue are not pushed around as roughly as with traditional lipo. Tumescent lipo also cuts down on blood loss, so we can safely remove even more fat. During the first few weeks, there is less post-operative swelling, bruising, and pain.

Ultrasound-Assisted Lipoplasty (UAL)

UAL relies on ultrasonic waves, transmitted beneath the skin through a wand-like device, to emulsify, or liquefy, the fat (whereas traditional lipo uses old-fashioned elbow-grease to break it up). The liquid fat actually flows out of each cell and is easy to suction out, reducing the trauma to the surrounding tissues. The blood vessels remain intact, so there is minimal bleeding. For obese individuals, large volumes of fat can be removed during a single procedure most conveniently using UAL.

External ultrasound is a variation of UAL. Instead of sound waves being delivered through a wand beneath the skin, a small, paddlelike box that generates radio waves is rubbed over the skin. This molds and changes the configuration of the fat cells to be suctioned, making them more pliable.

UAL is particularly effective when used on areas where fat is more fibrous, and also on connective tissue that is not just fat in such areas as the back, upper abdomen, arms, below the ribcage, and the male breast. Furthermore, UAL allows a continuous blood supply to flow to the skin, which means we can work "circumferentially"—on the front and back—during a single surgery without any danger.

Most of the risks associated with UAL are similar to those for traditional lipo, but there are others unique to the procedure. Since sound waves generate heat, there is a potential for burns to the skin and fat. (Another form of ultrasound, called Vaser, has recently been introduced, which uses a discontinuous pulse and therefore is less likely to burn.) UAL tends to take longer than traditional lipo because of the extra fat-liquefying step, and carries a greater risk of seroma, in which body fluid collects around the treated area (to avoid this, we may insert a temporary drain near the incision site to siphon off extra fluid). Because the process is labor-intensive and the equipment expensive, UAL typically costs more than other lipo techniques.

Power-Assisted Liposuction (PAL)

With this relatively new method, a machine causes the cannula to oscillate, allowing the surgeon to break up fat without having to exert great force. I use this technique more and more. There's no danger of burning, and it costs far less than UAL.

Endermologie

Endermologie, a nonsurgical technique that was invented in France in the 1970s, isn't actually liposuction, but some doctors use it with, or in place of, lipo. Endermologie claims to deal with the worst of all fat demons: cellulite. It allows electrical heating pulses to be shot through rollers that vigorously massage cellulite, and is repeated in weekly sessions. While there may be some evidence that pinching and squeezing tissue can break up the underlying fat, the benefits of Endermologie seem to be temporary and very costly. Until we have proof of long-term improvement, I don't recommend it.

URGENT QUESTION: *CAN LIPOSUCTION GET RID OF "COTTAGE-CHEESE" THIGHS?*

Cellulite isn't really fat: It's fibrous bands that connect skin to underlying muscle. The more inelastic skin gets, the more pronounced the cellulite. We can improve its appearance with liposuction by using a cannula directed at breaking up some of these fibrous bands, causing the tissue to heal in a different (and less lumpy) configuration. We might also use a "fat graft"—suctioning fat from one area and plumping up another—to smooth out the skin's surface. On the nonsurgical front, I have yet to hear of a cream that can convincingly tighten the skin for good; most of them temporarily improve cellulite's appearance by altering the water content in the fat cells. And while I'm wary of Endermologie's imperfect record of success, I'm encouraged by the development of techniques that use ultrasonic waves to break up these fibrous bands and redistribute them for a tighter, more uniform look.

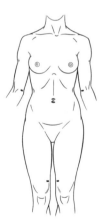

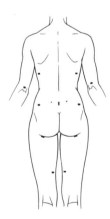

LIPOSUCTION SITES, INCLUDING NAVEL, ARM, AND INNER THIGHS

ADDITIONAL LIPO SITES, INCLUDING BACK, ARMS, BUTTOCKS, AND INNER THIGHS

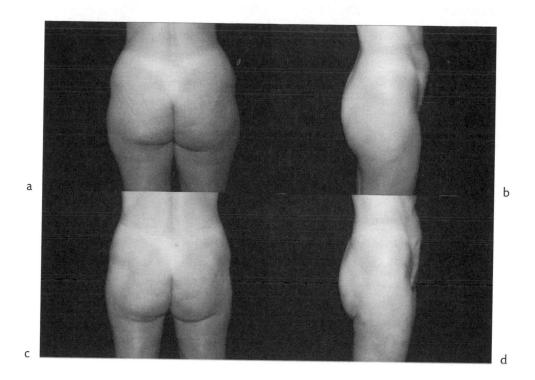

LIPOSUCTION TO THE ABDOMEN AND HIPS

Many women have trouble taking off the last few pounds of baby weight. This patient, thirty-one, gave birth a few months earlier, but was still unhappy with her 5'1", 132-pound shape. Despite regular exercise, the fat had collected primarily around her hips and thighs (a, b), and with the summer fast approaching she was eager to find a surgical solution to her problem. I performed liposuction on her trouble spots, removing close to five liters of fat, and the difference is obvious (c, d).

NECK-TO-ANKLE LIPOSUCTION

I use virtually all methods of liposuction, but in different combinations depending on a person's fat quality and the body part on which I'm working. Today, we can use liposuction to recontour the body from head to toe (or head to ankle, anyway). On which of these parts does liposuction work best, and when do you need to resort to a bigger recontouring procedure, such as a lift or tuck?

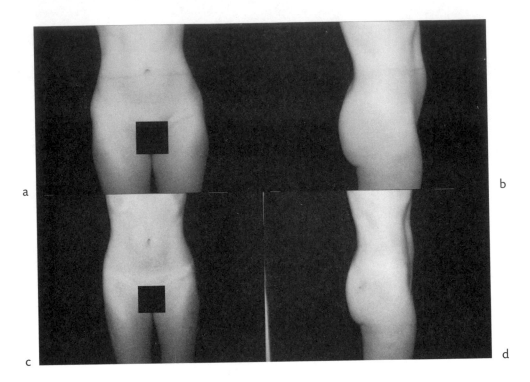

a

b

c

d

LIPO TO THE TUMMY, HIPS, AND THIGHS

You don't have to be "fat" to have liposuction. This thirty-five-year-old real estate broker worked out regularly, and though she was a relatively trim 117 pounds she felt she was carrying a little too much padding on her tummy, hips, and thighs (a, b). I did lipo in those spots, and eight months later she looks great (c, d)—not least because she became motivated to work out harder and lose even more weight once she was able to see her muscle definition again.

Abdomen and Hips

No amount of sit-ups can give you six-pack abs if the muscle is buried under layers of fat. An abdominoplasty (tummy tuck) used to be the only way to improve the midsection, but it leaves a hip-to-hip scar and requires a more arduous recovery. Through a tiny incision in the navel, liposuction sucks out the fat and eliminates a bulging tummy or love handles (see illustration at left on page 182), with virtually no downtime. When working on both a patient's front and sides, I find UAL and PAL to be especially effective.

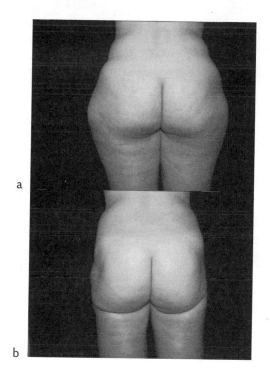

a

b

LIPO TO CORRECT HOURGLASS HIPS

No matter how much weight she lost or how many hours she logged at the gym, this twenty-six-year-old artistic program director just couldn't do anything to chisel away at her hourglass hips (a). Only 5'3" and 135 pounds, her deformity was exaggerated by her tiny waist. When she came to me, her goal was to be able to wear a narrow-fitting gown at her brother's wedding. I liposuctioned just over six liters of fat from her thighs and hips, using a combination of external and internal ultrasonic techniques. When I was done, she was a size six (b)!

Thighs

Lipo works beautifully to trim the outer thighs or dreaded "saddlebag" area. The incisions are placed above the bathing-suit line (high or low, depending on where yours falls) and the insides of the lower cheek crease (see illustrations on page 182). The inner thigh is trickier to fix than the outer, because the fat there tends to be fluffier and more prone to post-operative irregularities. But the skin on both sides of the thigh tightens

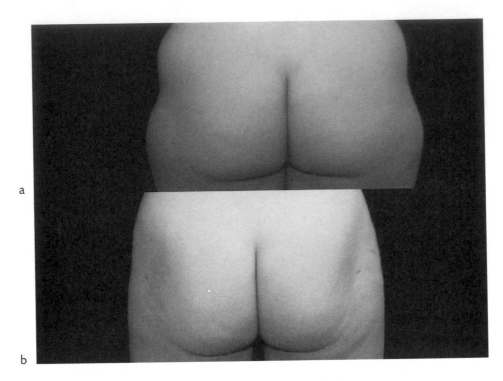

a

b

LIPO TO HIPS AND THIGHS

The "riding britches" deformity (a) is common in women, who tend to collect fat in and around their hips. This twenty-seven-year-old graphic designer had the pouches on her outer thighs and buttock area liposuctioned (about 2,000 cubic centimeters of fat). The scars are imperceptible—and what a difference to her figure (b).

beautifully after lipo, and the results are impressive when you consider the clunky alternative: a thighplasty, which requires a long incision around the leg and should therefore be done only as a last resort.

Arms

Lipo is the fastest way to say good-bye to fatty, wobbly arms. Usually, a tiny incision is made near the elbow (see illustrations on page 182) and the cannula is passed all the way up to the armpit. UAL and PAL are preferred methods for

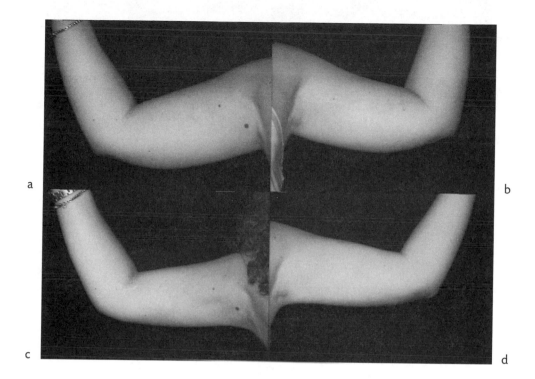

| a | b |
| c | d |

LIPO TO ARMS

Fleshy arms can make a woman look heavy, even if she isn't. That was the case with this twenty-six-year-old financial analyst, who, at 5'3" and 130 pounds had a cute figure but bulky arms (a, b). Through a tiny hole near each elbow, I liposuctioned out 700 cubic centimeters of fat from each arm—nearly a liter!—using a combination of external and internal ultrasound lipo, tumescent lipo, and PAL. Three months later she was wearing sleeveless tops, her scars virtually undetectable (c, d).

---

this, because fat tends to be tough there. If the arms are especially saggy, you may also need a brachioplasty, or arm lift, to get rid of excess skin.

Buttocks

We use liposuction in this area more and more: Through a quarter-inch incision in the hip or butt crease (discreetly hidden under your bathing-suit or underwear line, see illustration at right on page 182), fat is suctioned out to shrink the rear. To avoid "saggy butt" syndrome, we sometimes even *add back* fat to parts of the buttocks to recountour their whole shape. I tend to use UAL for this procedure, because the fat in this area can be fibrous and dense. If a patient's buttocks are too droopy, a last resort may be a buttock tuck to tighten the skin once excess fat is removed. However, a tuck leaves a big scar, making recovery quite literally a pain in the rear.

Breasts

Lipo (especially PAL) is an increasingly popular alternative to traditional breast reduction techniques: It's quick, and because the incision is made in the fold under the breasts, it leaves almost no scar. For best results, though, breasts need to be full, with good nipple position.

Neck and Jowls

There is a range of tightening options we commonly use to get rid of a turkey wattle or "tree-trunk" neck, all of which offer dramatic results. For a heavy neck that lacks definition, the fat can be liposuctioned out and the area slimmed through a tiny hole under the chin. Typically, however, the underlying platysma muscles (the cords that run up and down the front of the neck) are lax and therefore contribute to the problem. These muscles may be tightened through the same small incision in the chin. This procedure is called a **neck lipectomy.** The skin in this area tightens beautifully, and truthfully, no one will suspect you've had surgery. If, however, the skin is especially saggy around the neck and jowls, you may be better off combining liposuction with a **neck lift**, where the tissues and skin around the jawline are tightened through a small incision at the front of the ear. Your doctor will weigh the options based on your skin tone, facial contour, and desired results.

Back

Lipo in this area is especially popular among men, who struggle with lower-back fat and love handles. Many women, too, say they want to get rid of extra weight back there (it tends to deposit near the armpit) so that they can wear sleeveless shirts and sports bras more comfortably (see illustration at right on page 182). Because dorsal fat is fibrous, UAL and PAL allow us to recontour the back in a way that we never could before.

Calves

Women who hide their "table legs" under long skirts, take heart: Calves are highly malleable using a very fine cannula and the smallest of incisions—usually one near the ankle and one in the back of the leg. Because of the elasticity of skin there, results tend to be very good. However, recovery time can be prolonged, since gravity, especially when you're sitting, promotes swelling.

Ankles and Knees

Lipo easily reduces the bulge in both these areas, and the skin typically retracts well. The incisions are easily hidden in the body's natural contours: at the front of the knee, in the crease at the back of the knee, and on the side of the ankle. Because a procedure on such bony body parts requires delicacy, we typically rely on traditional lipo using tiny cannulas. Again, recovery time tends to be longer than average because of gravity's effect on swelling.

Enlarged Male Breasts

Otherwise known as **gynecomastia**, this mostly genetic condition results in swollen breasts that can be embarrassing, even emotionally debilitating, for men (for more on this procedure, see Chapter 11). Today, it's very easy to reduce male breast size through a tiny incision at the edge of the areola; UAL and PAL are particularly effective in this area, as the fat tends to be fibrous.

PREPARING FOR LIPOSUCTION

As with all surgeries, avoid spicy or salty foods and alcohol the day before the procedure to limit the risk of swelling. For two weeks prior to surgery, do not take aspirin or anti-inflammatory medications, which inhibit clotting. For more information on preparation and recovery, see Chapter 12. A few specifics:

◆ Do not show up for surgery with a new suntan or sunburn. Sun stresses the skin and compromises healing; you may also end up with inconsistencies in pigmentation in the affected area as the skin contracts and tightens.

◆ Bring comfortable clothing that you can put on easily after surgery, such as a button-down shirt and loose-fitting pants.

◆ Shower the night before, since you won't be able to do so again for the first post-operative week.

◆ A special note for men: If you're having abdominal liposuction, bring a jockstrap for support to wear after the operation.

What the Surgery Involves

Lipo isn't called the "quick fix" for nothing. Almost all procedures take only an hour or so to perform. They are typically done in an office operating room, using only local anesthesia and twilight sedation. Patients walk out afterward without feeling groggy, and often may return to their normal lives the next day.

For starters, your surgeon will likely indicate with a pen the spot(s) to be treated. This works as a guide for the doctor to know exactly where and how much to suction. During this process the patient stands upright, because fat shifts and sinks when you lie down. The most fat I remove in a single lipo procedure (which varies depending on the part of the body or face being lipoed) is eight to ten pounds, which is far below the point at which complications generally develop. Where possible, your surgeon should make an effort to conceal incisions in natural skin creases—the bottom of the buttocks, the navel, the pubic area, the back of the knee, the nipple—and suture *under* the skin to minimize scarring.

The surgeon will insert the cannula, and start breaking up and suctioning the fat. It's physical work; we actually burn hundreds of calories while doing it! The surgeon moves the cannula through different depths of fat, in different directions, alternately removing superficial and deep fat so that there's an even distribution in the area. The yellowish, jellylike fat, along with blood and other fluids, flows through the tube, gets sucked into a canister, and is disposed of. Near the end of the process, thinner cannulas are used for sculpting superficial fat. The incision is then sewn shut and dressed. Depending on the lipo performed, your surgeon may put in drains—tubes with little reservoirs to collect fluid—for twenty-four to seventy-two hours.

LIPO TO GO?

A handful of surgeons today is promoting a form of liposuction that's so convenient you don't even need to lie down on an operating table. Called "walking" or "standing" liposuction, its practitioners claim that it allows them to better assess where the fat needs to be extracted because the doctor can see where it "naturally" falls, thanks to gravity. I find this preposterous. As quick and easy as liposuction seems, it's surgery, not the McDonald's drive-thru. Your body can't sustain a heavy volume change, or effectively maintain blood flow to your extremities, when you're on your feet. A good surgeon can tell how your anatomy changes from lying down, to sitting, to standing, and will be able to remove the fat in the right amounts, and from the right areas, when you're flat on your back, side, or stomach.

Recovery

For the most part, recovery from liposuction is easily manageable. Since clothing can conceal areas that have been sculpted, most patients are back at work after just a couple of days.

During your first week, you'll need to wear a tight-fitting elastic compression garment to help the skin adhere to the underlying muscle and remaining fat, and also to keep things from shifting around. In short, this garment helps to define your new body shape. (Some patients say it feels like wearing a girdle or a wet suit.) The garment also helps to prevent fluid from collecting under the skin, compresses the incisions together, and reduces swelling. At a week to ten days, you can remove the garment to shower, though you'll likely have to wear it for an additional week. You may decide you want to even if not required: After a few days it becomes something of a security blanket, and some patients find they never want to take it off!

Common Side Effects

Although recovery from liposuction is generally quite smooth, there are a few side effects to be aware of:

Swelling and Bruising
Normal puffiness will resolve over a couple of weeks; typically, swelling affects the lower extremities more than other parts of the body. At the lipo sites, bruising may linger for up to three weeks.

Bumps and Lumps
Fat needs time to shift into position, and sometimes the scar tissue doesn't form evenly. This is the limitation of lipo: Since no skin is removed, tightening can be a bit unpredictable, and irregularities in contour can occur. But massage helps smooth these imperfections, and if an area is particularly lumpy, we can improve it with another procedure such as external ultrasound—or, as a last resort, corrective surgery.

Hypersensitivity
You may experience hypersensitivity around the sites that have been liposuctioned; this typically subsides within a few weeks. You should not feel severe pain. If you do, contact your surgeon.

Numbness

Since nerves may be temporarily damaged during surgery, you may experience a loss of sensation at or around the lipo sites. "Even after the swelling goes down there's a tingling kind of pain, as if something has fallen asleep," recalls one patient. Massage can help improve the condition; only very rarely is this symptom permanent.

Scars

The great thing about the incisions used for liposuction is that they're tiny and discreetly placed. If you're someone whose scars tend to keloid (become red and "angry"), however, this may indeed happen. To help reduce the risk, I give patients a steroid cream and scar gel to help smooth out the scars during the healing process.

Hyperpigmentation

Any time you stimulate the skin to regenerate or tighten, it may produce too much or too little pigment. You can even out skin tone using topical creams and glycolic acids.

Stiffness

Some patients are so conscientious about remaining still after the procedure that they develop neck, shoulder, or back stiffness. This is easily prevented by staying moderately mobile.

A week or so after surgery, I have my patients start to work out with a trainer. Light exercise is terrific for the healing process, as it boosts circulation and stimulates the skin to tighten. Don't do anything that will cause you to sweat in your compressive garment, though: It can increase the risk of infection. After three weeks, most patients can resume more strenuous aerobic exercise. When bruising disappears, you can even start weight training. The psychological boost and endorphin high you get from exercise are, in my opinion, at least as important as the physical benefits.

Side Effects to Be Concerned About

Liposuction can be performed on almost any body part. But some parts are more forgiving than others, and each person's body "settles" and sculpts differently. Depending on your healing abilities, the skill of the surgeon, the area(s) being treated, and other criteria, there are always potential complications, including:

Contour Irregularities

After the swelling subsides, you may notice dimpling, rippling, bagginess, and lumpiness in the lipoed areas. These imperfections may be improved with massage, topical creams, or external ultrasound, but if they persist, a follow-up procedure like a fat injection can be effective.

Asymmetry

We try to calculate precisely how much fat to remove from a site, but each side of the body is a different size and shape, and sometimes the results aren't totally balanced. If necessary, more fat can be removed (or added back) in a follow-up procedure.

Permanent Discoloration

Though the hyperpigmentation usually fades within a few months, it may become permanent if skin is exposed to too much sun either before or after surgery.

Loss of Sensation

In extremely rare cases, numbness can last for months or become permanent if nerves have been damaged in the surgery.

BUYER BEWARE: UNLICENSED LIPO

In the last few years there has been much publicity about a handful of liposuction cases that resulted in severe complications. Because lipo is so quick and offers instant results, lots of non–plastic surgeons are performing it.

Although the procedure seems easy, *it is surgery*. Many of these new practitioners aren't even trained M.D.s and are shockingly unprepared to deal with complications should they arise. In some notorious instances, death has resulted when too much fat was removed. Although technically you can remove as much fat as you want, a large volume shift could send the patient into shock, which can be fatal. When patients need more than about twelve pounds removed, we simply perform a second surgery later.

Furthermore, many of the folks who just hang out a liposuction shingle, be it at a spa, health club, or private office, are practicing in terribly unsanitary conditions, without masks, gloves, lab coat, or even a dedicated operating room. An unsterile environment greatly increases your risk of infection. For your own safety, you must insist that your surgeon perform in a licensed operating room (see Chapter 4 for more information on how to find out whether a surgical facility is licensed).

Patience, Patient

Lipo is great for instant-gratification seekers: If you were a size 10 before, it's conceivable that within a few days of surgery you'll find yourself trying on size 6 or 8 clothing. But don't fret if you still see imperfections in your shape several weeks later. It can take four months, even a year, to get an accurate picture of how the body will look once the swelling subsides and everything settles into place. "At first there wasn't a huge difference in my appearance. In fact, I seemed bigger because of the swelling," recalls Alyssa, the med student. "Then, about four months later, I suddenly felt very skinny and people started commenting on my weight loss." Lipo patients who started out especially overweight will have to bide their time before realizing their dream results, because it takes several weeks for skin to redrape over the new area and for tissue to heal completely.

You should be able to maintain your new shape with basic exercise and diet maintenance. Even if you gain weight, it will distribute more evenly, instead of accumulating in former trouble zones. The good news is that so many of my patients use the occasion of their cosmetic surgery, particularly lipo, to springboard to better health habits. Maybe it's the confidence they get from no longer having to worry about embarassingly outsized arms or hips or stomach, or maybe it's a feeling of responsibility to their new, improved selves. The lipo may give patients a little bit of a "free pass," but almost invariably they use it as an occasion to make their bodies and entire lifestyles much healthier—to start, with great enthusiasm, down the road of cosmetic wellness.

LIFTS AND TUCKS: WHEN LIPO ISN'T ENOUGH

Sucking out fat from a chronic problem area may be all you need to look firmer and more toned. But what if it doesn't go far enough? Sometimes, after a significant amount of fat has been removed, the skin covering that area sags, making you appear even older and less fit than you looked before. This droopy "excess" skin may result from a number of factors:

- age
- pregnancy (especially multiple pregnancies or carrying a large child)
- obesity
- significant and/or repeated weight gain and loss
- genes (some people's skin has more give to it, even when young)

Even tissues *underneath* the skin can sag. Exercise has little or no effect on muscles (abs, for example) that may have stretched due to weight loss or pregnancy, and a thousand sit-ups a day won't get them to retract normally. If weight loss and/or lipo don't, by themselves, help you achieve the firmer look you dreamed of, then the solution may be to tighten the skin with either a lift or a tuck (think "lift up" and "tuck down"). These skin reduction techniques, in conjunction with liposuction, comprise the methods for body recontouring.

In a lift or a tuck, an incision is made, the underlying fat is removed through liposuction, muscles are tightened, and the remaining skin is lifted or pulled to firm up the area. The newly redraped skin is sutured into place until it heals.

However, there's a trade-off for the dramatic physical improvement brought about by a lift or tuck: a big scar. There's just no way (right now, anyway) to camouflage a scar when you excise large amounts of skin. Nonetheless, a scar may be a small price to pay for the person whose skin has been the very thing preventing him or her from leading a normal life.

A New Body, A New Life

When Jessica came to me nearly two years ago, she was already a shadow of her former self. A forty-three-year-old schoolteacher, she had struggled with her weight her entire life and in recent years peaked at about 250 pounds. "I had tried every diet in the book," she recalls, despairingly. "Each time, I would lose my standard twenty-five pounds, but after that my weight wouldn't budge." What motivated Jessica to seek a surgical solution—bariatric surgery, more commonly known as "stomach stapling"—was the recognition that she was dealing with a disease—obesity—and not just a cosmetic issue. "Society makes you feel as if you should be able to lose weight, even large amounts, on your own," she continues. "Not only *couldn't* I do it on my own, but ninety-nine percent of people couldn't have done it, either. All the willpower in the world wasn't going to make a difference. I had a medical problem, and I needed a medical solution."

As a result of her stomach surgery a year earlier, Jessica had dropped about 100 pounds, and by the time she walked into my office she was well on her way to losing more. She was thrilled with her shape, which now allowed her to exercise, shop, work, and generally live her life with greater ease and confidence. But there was a problem: She had several pounds of loose skin draping her body. Fat supports the skin, and once the fat had vanished there was nothing left to hold the skin up. Jessica was nervous about seeing a plastic surgeon; she knew the doctor would ask her to get naked and then scrutinize every inch of her. I tried to make her feel comfortable by not being excessively physical, and encouraging her to collaborate on deciding what surgeries she should have, and in what order.

Jessica really felt that her whole body needed lifting—her arms, breasts, abdomen, back, and thighs. But it would be medically risky, if not impossible, to do everything at once. Since she was planning on losing even more weight, we decided to stage her operations to improve first the areas that most concerned her and that would be minimally affected by further weight loss. We also decided to spread the surgeries over the period of a year so she would miss as little work as possible.

I began by lifting Jessica's breasts and arms, since they could be worked on at the same time. A couple of months later, during her summer vacation, I performed a tummy tuck; this had to be done before the thighs and back were addressed, because the thighs would have to be lifted up to the hip area. Once her weight stabilized, we would work our way to the lower body.

Today Jessica is 134 pounds, and a size 6 or 8. She insists that it's as if her life has started over again:

> *"My ability to just plain feel good inside my body increased even more after having plastic surgery. I fell in love with yoga, and I'm planning to start a salsa aerobics class soon. And the clothes! I love clothes now, and I have a lot of them. When you're a heavy woman in today's society, you tend to buy clothes because they fit you—you buy them large, loose, dark, and accessorize with jewelry and scarves to make yourself look attractive. Big clothes are also expensive. Now shopping is so much fun: I can even buy off the sale rack at Banana Republic! One of my greatest victories has to do with this beautiful pair of cowboy boots that I ordered out of a catalog a few years ago. When they arrived, they didn't fit me because my calves were too big. But I kept them anyway, and now I can finally wear them."*

The surgeries have allowed Jessica to make enormous progress in the confidence department. "The scars are finally fading," she says. "With the weight loss I felt really good about my body *in* clothes, and now I'm getting to the point where I can feel good about my body *out* of clothes."

These positive changes to Jessica's outlook have begun to make themselves felt in her professional life, too:

> *"As an educator, I'm in a line of work where I could get by pretty well looking as I used to. There are lots of heavy people in the school system. But I have*

noticed a new dynamic in the way people treat me, especially men. I received two job offers this week, and I'm not even doing a job search. A hundred and twenty pounds ago, that wouldn't have happened. I really do believe in better living through surgery. Of course, I wish we lived in a world where there was greater acceptance for all body types. But if there are solutions that can help us not to suffer, to feel at peace and in harmony with our bodies, then that's a good thing."

Most patients who need body recontouring will not require a full body lift, like Jessica had, or even a lift in more than one area. It was just a handful of years ago, however, that the kind of transformation Jessica underwent was impossible because of the risk to one's health. Fortunately, we're always making advances in the science of skin reduction—incisions are smaller, fat removal is easier, and "mini" procedures have supplanted the once-obligatory full ones.

Next I'll discuss the most commonly performed lift-and-tuck procedures, and who makes a good candidate for each. At the end of the chapter, I'll deal with recovery and risks for all procedures.

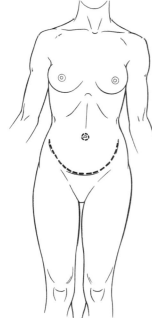

TUMMY TUCK
INCISION

Abdominoplasty (Tummy Tuck)

It used to be that a tuck was the only option for a woman with a bulging tummy. Then lipo came along, and we could do a smaller procedure with no scarring. However, people who have especially slack skin in their midsection need more than what lipo can offer. Typical candidates for this surgery are women with drooping abdomens after pregnancy, women and men who've lost a great deal of weight or who have lost and gained weight repeatedly, menopausal women, and older people with loose skin due to age. In a tummy tuck, the skin from the rib cage down to the pelvic area is tightened, and the navel is moved up and secured in a new position.

QUOTE, UNQUOTE

"During my first pregnancy, I put on nearly 70 pounds even though I was conscientious about eating. During my second pregnancy, I vowed not to let that happen again. Well, it didn't matter what I ate. I ballooned to more than 200 pounds! Once I felt strong enough, I went on a strict protein diet and started exercising vigorously for the first time in my life. All the pregnancy weight melted away—and then some. In fact, I hadn't been so thin since before college. The only problem was I now had all this horrible-looking, dark skin hanging down from my stomach over my underwear. It was devastating. While my husband continued to tell me he thought I looked beautiful, I just didn't *feel* beautiful. I had to hide my stomach by wearing loose pants and baggy shirts and sweaters, even at the beach! After my tummy tuck, I felt instantly lighter and more agile. When the garment came off, I cried. That heavy skin was gone, and I could see the abs I'd worked so hard to develop in the previous few months. Now I'm training for a marathon and find I can run so much faster and more comfortably without the bulk."

—Betsy, 32-year-old mother of two

PREPARING FOR A TUCK

As with any surgery, avoid salty and spicy foods the day before because they can raise blood pressure; also, steer clear of aspirin and anti-inflammatories, which can inhibit blood clotting. A couple of special tips for patients getting ready for a tummy tuck or a buttock, thigh, or arm lift:

◆ On the day of surgery, wear loose-fitting clothing that won't constrict your incisions or force you to bend your legs (if you've had work on the lower half) or raise your arms (if you're having a brachioplasty).

◆ Avoid the sun for at least one week before surgery. Sun stresses skin, reducing its resiliency and ability to heal. Moreover, increased pigmentation in the skin leaves the tuck area vulnerable to color irregularities.

◆ If your abdominal walls are being tightened, your doctor may have you do a "cleanout" of the bowels the day before using a mild laxative.

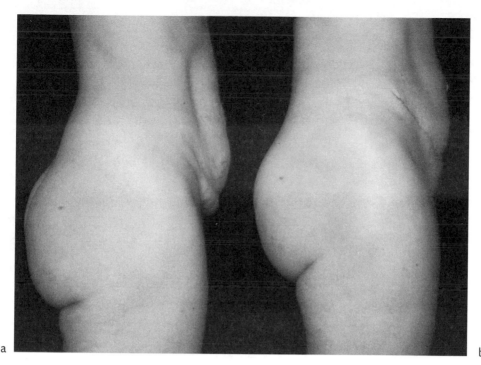

a   b

TUMMY TUCK

Pregnancy can really do a number on the abdomen. This thirty-one-year-old mother of two was—at 5'5" and 137 pounds—in very good physical shape, but her abdominal skin sagged dramatically and she had terrible stretch marks above and below her navel (a). These deformities made her a perfect candidate for a tummy tuck. Making an incision just above her pubic area, I removed the skin below her navel (and with it, a good deal of her stretch marks), pulled down the skin from above, and repositioned the navel in a new spot (b). Her scar, though prominent, will be completely hidden by her underwear or bathing suit.

When planning a tummy tuck, an enlightened surgeon will want to know the favorite bathing suit you plan to wear after recovery. The shape of your suit can help the doctor decide where to put the incisions. A tummy tuck is usually done under twilight sedation and local anesthesia, though many doctors still prefer to use general anesthesia due to the extensiveness of this operation. The surgeon typically makes a slightly rounded, horizontal incision from one hip to the other, just above the pubic area (the shape depends on your anatomy; some surgeons prefer a 'W'). Another incision is made around the navel, to allow the bellybutton to be loosened from the surrounding tissue (see illustration on page 199). The surgeon then separates the skin from the abdominal wall to which it's attached and lifts this flap away from the abdomen, all the way up to the rib cage. He or she will pull together any loose or stretched abdominal muscles and suture them to keep them from sagging. (This also helps to narrow the waistline.) Liposuction is used to remove fat pockets, and then the skin is pulled down tight over the abdomen and the excess is cut away, yielding a beautiful, flat stomach. Women with unsightly stretch marks in the lower abdomen will be thrilled to find that these are eliminated; unfortunately, if stretch marks extend to the upper abdomen, we generally can't remove them. Finally, the newly positioned navel is reconstructed and, if need be, reshaped.

The surgery takes three-plus hours; if you're having the procedure as an outpatient, you'll be able to go home shortly thereafter. You can generally return to work in two weeks. Note that you may walk and sit a little hunched over for a few days after the operation. Don't even try to stand up straight during this time—you risk separating the incisions. Also, you should minimize the strenuousness or suddenness of such exertions as coughing, sneezing, laughing, and bowel movements.

URGENT QUESTION: *CAN I STILL HAVE CHILDREN AFTER A TUMMY TUCK?*

What if you get pregnant after an abdominoplasty? Not long ago, if you had your abdominal walls tightened, it was recommended that you not get pregnant again because of the increased risk (wholly speculative) of miscarriage. While it doesn't make much sense to tighten things only to have pregnancy loosen them again, you can, post-tuck, become pregnant and bring a healthy baby to term. But if you are fairly certain that you want to have more kids, you should discuss this issue with your surgeon.

MINI-ABDOMINOPLASTY
(MINI–TUMMY TUCK)

The mini–tummy tuck is a great option for those who want to slim the stomach and waist but don't need the heavy lifting of a full abdominoplasty. It's especially effective for those who suffer from a moderate but persistent potbelly or "bikini bulge," but who look pretty good from the navel up. The main difference between the two procedures is that the mini–tummy tuck doesn't require moving or reconstructing the navel.

This procedure is typically done today under twilight sedation and local anesthesia, though some doctors still opt to use general anesthesia. The surgeon will make a small incision near the navel to liposuction out the fat in the abdominal area. He or she will then make an incision from one side of the pelvis to the other (shorter than the one made in a full tummy tuck); if necessary, tighten the muscles of the abdominal wall from the pubic region to the navel; and remove the excess skin in the abdomen area. Since the skin above the navel isn't being pulled down, as in a full tummy tuck, the navel will stay where it is.

The surgery takes roughly an hour and a half. Since the mini–tummy tuck, as its name suggests, is limited in scope, recovery is quicker than for a full abdominoplasty—between five days and two weeks, depending on how much the muscles were tightened.

THE MARK OF ZORRO: BIG SCARS

I don't want to frighten you, but most lifts leave you with unsightly scars. There are many things surgeons do to improve a scar's appearance. Today, we suture almost every incision *under* the skin, leaving no stitch marks or "railroad tracks." Working with the patient, a surgeon can also best determine the positioning of most scars. Before surgery, find out what kind of sutures your doctor favors: Some use traditional sutures, some staples, some dissolving sutures (my preference); some sew under the skin, others over. Each technique and suture material results in a different-looking scar. Over time, the scar will flatten out. But I also strongly recommend "working" scars with ointments such as steroid creams, silicone gels, and pigment blockers, which soften and improve the coloration of the area. The willingness to follow this regimen has, in my patients, brought about quick, positive results in keeping scars smooth, inconspicuous, and relatively pliable. For more information on scar formation and healing, see Chapter 12.

BUTTOCK LIFT

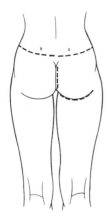

**BUTTOCK LIFT
INCISION**

You don't need me to tell you that the derrière is a tremendously sensuous part of the body. In James Joyce's classic novel *Ulysses*, Leopold Bloom rhapsodizes about his wife Molly's behind as the turn-on to end all turn-ons ("melonous smellonous osculations"). When the backside goes, though, it's not a pretty sight, whether it's the kind that sags or the one that's pocked by cellulite. The buttock lift is a big operation that leaves a long scar, and it can have a difficult recovery if the incision is made under the rear (rather than at the waist), since the patient will not be able to sit down for several days. I tend to avoid this surgery, and opt instead for a combination of liposuction and fat grafts to round out the buttocks and get rid of sagginess. Sometimes, though, if there is too much excess skin in this area, a buttock lift is the only procedure likely to bring satisfactory results.

This procedure is now most often performed under twilight sedation with local anesthesia, but some doctors still prefer general anesthesia. Many surgeons make the incisions just under each cheek, where the scars will be most discreet; I try, if possible, to make them at the waist or even in the crack of the buttocks so patients are able to sit down without too much pain (see illustration). Typically, liposuction is performed first, to reduce the buttocks' size. Sometimes, though, fat is added back to plump up the rear and prevent "pancaking." The remaining skin is either pulled down and sutured to the crease just under the cheek or lifted up to the waist. This surgery lasts three to four hours; expect to be out from work for two to three weeks.

THIGHPLASTY

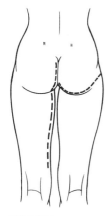

**THIGHPLASTY
INCISION**

I personally resort to this operation *only* when liposuction falls short of a solution. Again, I'm hesitant to perform it because the groin area heals slowly and patients are left with a big scar (which most surgeons try to hide under the bathing suit area). But if trimming your "saddlebags" with lipo is going to leave the skin saggier than before, or if your skin is very loose to begin with, especially from high-volume weight loss, a thighplasty may be the only answer.

Using twilight sedation and local anesthesia, your surgeon will typically make an incision in the groin crease in front of the body and continue around the inner thigh to the buttock crease (see illustration). If both inner and outer thighs are being lifted, the incision may encircle the leg or run vertically from the knee to the groin. The surgeon will then suction out fat from the thighs. Next, the skin on the front and sides of the thighs is lifted and tightened, along with the underlying connective tissue. The skin is then sutured into its new, taut position.

The surgery takes three to five hours or more, and the patient is turned over several times during the procedure. Mobility will be quite limited during your recovery, which lasts between two and three weeks (sitting upright may be out of the question for a few days).

Is a thighplasty right for you? Consider whether it's the sagging or volume of your thighs that bothers you more. If it's their volume, liposuction—a quick procedure with a fast recovery and virtually no scars—is the way to go (and lipo does result in some tightening of the skin). If the skin is very loose, however, a thighplasty will undoubtedly give you a better result, so long as you don't mind the resulting scars.

BRACHIOPLASTY (ARMLIFT)

Lifts on this famously wobbly part of the human physiognomy—known familiarly as "Hi Janes" or "Bingo" arms—are particularly popular. Heavy and even

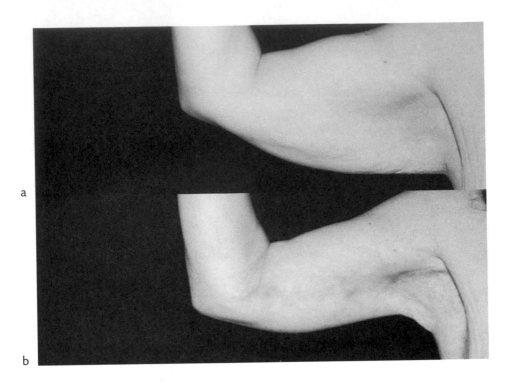

a

b

BRACHIOPLASTY

I did an arm lift on this patient's arms (b). Liposuction wouldn't have been enough, since her skin was too loose to tighten on its own (a).

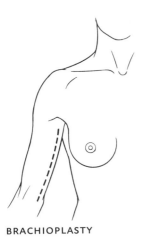

BRACHIOPLASTY
INCISION

moderately droopy arms can be recontoured very effectively with liposuction. But if a patient is left with severely hanging skin as a result of age or weight loss, a brachioplasty will be the most effective procedure—though once again, the trade-off for tightness is a big scar.

Today an arm lift procedure takes a relatively quick two to three hours, typically under twilight sedation and local anesthesia. Your surgeon will need to make a considerable incision, nearly a foot long from armpit to elbow (see illustration). The excess fat is sucked out using liposuction, the underlying connective tissues are tightened, extra skin is removed, and the skin is sutured into place. Your mobility isn't as restricted as after a lower-body lift, and many patients find they can return to work after a week. Do not, however, carry heavy bags, attempt any upper-body exercise, or raise your arms over your head (that Bruce Springsteen concert is probably out).

FULL BODY LIFT

Everything hangs: The chest, breasts, stomach, pubic area, sides of the waist. Today we can lift every part of a person's anatomy, as I did with Jessica though not all at once. Doing so would put your health in jeopardy, causing dangerous fluctuations in blood pressure and metabolism, as well as raising the risk of infection. Instead, your doctor will stage the operation, beginning with the body part or parts that are most bothersome to you or that follow a natural progression. It makes most medical sense, for instance, to begin lifting from top to bottom, as gravity's pull will affect how the lower surgeries turn out. It will be up to your doctor whether to go from back to front, or vice versa.

In cases where more than one surgery is combined—in Jessica's case, breast and arm lifts, though the abdominal lift and back lift are also routinely done together—a doctor may decide to start work on a patient's back or sides, since the patient will be unable to be prone after surgery. The patient is then turned over and the next surgery is completed. Although I swear by twilight sedation and local anesthesia, plenty of doctors opt to use general anesthesia or spinal epidurals for a body lift because the combined surgeries can be fairly extensive.

LIFTS AND TUCKS: RECOVERY SCENARIOS

Since any procedure that involves the removal of skin constitutes major surgery, it is imperative that you have someone at home to wait on you for at least the first twenty-four hours, if not to assist for the first week—to help you get around, to eat, to go to the bathroom, and, most important, to lift things.

For the first two weeks, as with liposuction, you will need to wear a tight-fitting elastic compression garment to help the skin re-attach to the underlying muscle and remaining fat and to keep things from shifting, so you don't

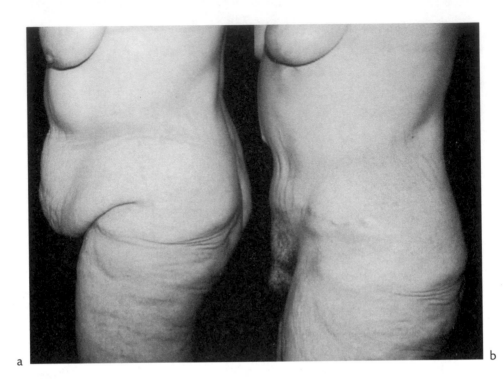

a   b

FULL BODY LIFT

Full-body lifts are rare, but I do them in the event of massive weight loss. This forty-three-year-old schoolteacher shed more than 100 pounds as a result of a stomach-stapling operation. When she came to me, her skin draped over her body like a blanket. It wasn't just ugly; it prevented her from exercising to lose even more weight (a). We decided to perform a series of lifts, staging them so that none would necessitate her being hospitalized and she could return to work between surgeries. First I did a breast lift. A few weeks later, I got rid of the "apron" of skin on her belly with a tummy tuck (b). In a few months we'll do her back and legs. While the patient will have fairly prominent scars in those areas, they are a worthwhile trade-off for a body that looks infinitely more youthful and retains no suggestion of her former obesity.

suffer major contour irregularities. This garment helps define your new body shape by pressing the skin together while it adheres. The garment also helps to prevent fluid from collecting under the skin and reduces swelling. (Fortunately, you can camouflage it under loose clothing.)

Most people return to work within two weeks of surgery. If you push yourself too hard, however, you can get an infection or complicate the healing process. Strenuous activities from exercise to lifting bags of groceries are strictly forbidden for at least four weeks post-op. Any increase in blood pressure ups your risk for hematoma. Seroma, or a pooling of fluid under the skin, is also a possibility. To minimize the risk, your doctor will probably put drains (fluid-collecting reservoirs) at the incision sites for twenty-four to seventy-two hours.

How much pain will you feel? Individual experiences vary. You may feel very little, or you may experience intense pain for at least two days, which is more likely the case if you've had muscles tightened (you'll probably want to take a prescription anti-inflammatory medication and a painkiller).

Common Side Effects and Their Treatment

Blood and Fluid Leakage

Drains will be placed at the incision sites to siphon off liquid; accumulation should stop within a couple of days.

Tightness and/or Discomfort

You may experience a bit to a lot of discomfort, and even pain, after a lift or a tuck, especially where muscles have been tightened and/or removed. Expect to be on pain medication for several days.

Bruising and Swelling

This will be most apparent around the incisions and can be managed, in part, with anti-inflammatories. The swelling may last a month or longer.

Loss of Sensation

Numbness around the incisions and in areas where muscles have been tightened is not unusual. The condition should be temporary, but may last as long as six months while nerve function returns to normal.

Scar Irritation

The incisions can be painful as they heal. Do not touch them until the stitches are either removed or have dissolved; even then, keep the area very clean. As the scar flattens and becomes less red and tender it may itch; cortisone cream can help relieve this (ask your doctor before applying).

Hematoma

The risk of blood accumulating under the skin increases as a result of vigorous activity or lifting. Take it easy for at least the first week after surgery.

Seroma

Fluid can accumulate under the skin within the first couple of days after surgery. These collections can be drained with a needle and are not harmful.

Side Effects to Be Concerned About

Embolism

Blood clots can form in the legs and travel to the lungs. This is a serious condition. If you feel shortness of breath, swelling or pain in the lower leg, or chest pain, contact your doctor right away.

Lymphodema

When the lymphatic system is traumatized during surgery, it doesn't drain properly. To open up the lymphatics and reduce swelling, I encourage all patients to return for a lymphatic massage within a week or two of surgery. Elevation of the affected area also curtails the effects of lymphodema.

Asymmetry

It's not a perfect world. With a tummy tuck, scarring may pull the navel too far to one side; with a butt lift, one buttock may end up slightly smaller than the other. It's likely that the imperfection is perceptible only to you. If there's a real problem, however, we can usually correct it with a follow-up procedure.

Keloidal Scars

All lifts and tucks leave a significant scar. Scars should flatten and regular color should return within a few months of surgery, but some people are more prone to hypertrophied scars, or those in which there is an overproduction of cells. Some scars can even develop keloids (become red and fiery, or, in ethnic skins, grow darker than the surrounding skin); their appearance can be improved with steroid creams, steroid injections, laser treatment, and pigment-blocking cream.

Permanent Numbness

It is possible for a nerve to be severed in surgery, resulting in a permanent loss of sensation either at the incision site or around the area that has been lifted.

Skin Death

If you smoke or have poor circulation, you are at heightened risk for skin death after surgery, since the blood flow to the skin's surface is compromised. The resulting wound may heal by itself in the following weeks or may require a follow-up procedure to fix.

Infection

As with any surgery, there's a small risk of infection at the site of the wound. If the scar becomes very red and full of pus, and/or you have a fever, your incision may be infected and you must call your doctor.

Recontouring techniques are only going to become more advanced and exciting in the future. For now liposuction, combined with traditional lifts and tucks, is the closest we surgeons get to being able to wave a magic wand at your body and reshape the parts you'd like to live without.

11

Men: Same Idea, Different Procedures

When Geoff, a thirty-nine-year-old, tired-looking, slightly overweight insurance executive, came to see me a year ago, he was looking to shrink his thick midsection. "I have a hereditary tendency to gain weight just in my stomach," he told me. "My arms, butt, and face all look normal, but my stomach—oof! It just hangs out there." Geoff had never even heard of liposuction, the quick and relatively risk-free way of sucking out body fat. Within minutes, he was sold on the idea—and more. He asked if I thought there was any other part of his body that could benefit from lipo. I pointed out that his double chin could easily be eliminated that way; with just a little tightening of the underlying muscle, he could regain definition he'd no doubt had in his youth. To my surprise, Geoff signed on for that procedure, too, and didn't stop there.

"What else, doc?" he kept asking. "I'm here, so I might as well get a total makeover." We decided to remove some puffiness around his eyes, which also bore dark rings, making him look exhausted. He was especially excited about that procedure; he'd had no idea there was anything to be done about his "raccoon-eye" problem.

Today, after abdominal liposuction, a neck lipectomy, and an eyelid lift, Geoff looks more than a decade younger than he used to. Here's what he says:

"After the operations, I decided to go in for LASIK surgery on my eyes as well, so I could toss out the glasses I'd been wearing for years. Now I find that most of my customers do a double-take. The other day, an older lady came into the office with a question and hesitated before presenting her case. 'I bought my insurance policy from your father,' she said, scrutinizing my face. 'No, ma'am,' I answered. 'That was me.' She insisted: 'No, he was older, heavier, and he wore glasses.' That's when I knew I'd done the right thing."

Geoff is one of dozens of men who have walked through my door in the last couple of years. Men now comprise between 10 and 15 percent of my practice, whereas just a few years ago it was roughly 5 percent. Why are their ranks growing—not just in my practice, but nationally? (Since 1997, according to the ASAPS, there has been a 256-percent increase in procedures performed on men.) And why is it now acceptable for men to care about their looks?

I have a few theories. First, along with women, men are working longer and need to maintain a more youthful appearance. The tired look produced by sagging skin (exacerbated by those extra pounds), droopy lids, and heavy scowl lines can suggest that you're no longer a vital contributor. Second, many successful, results-driven men have more disposable income to use on something they've secretly wanted (in a couple of hours, you can rid yourself of decades-old love handles, get a stronger chin, lift those eyelids, or add a sexy suggestion of muscle to that chest). Third, men are getting married later, and getting remarried later. And fourth, many men (still) marry women who are considerably younger. For all these reasons, men no longer tiptoe toward the idea of plastic surgery but have started to embrace it as a quick, efficient, proven way to look better. "I'm conscious of what people think of me, so I certainly don't advertise the fact that I've had liposuction," says one of my male patients. "But I do think that if more guys like me knew about it, they'd opt to do the same thing."

The medical and technical advances in surgery I've discussed throughout this book are especially great for men. Small incisions make it easier to perform certain procedures like face and eyebrow lifts on patients with thinning or no hair, because the resulting scars are so much smaller than those left by the traditional face-lift that was the sole option a few years back. Also, many of the newest procedures have a very brief recovery time—and men notoriously resist resting.

Ultimately, though, plastic surgery's draw is its results. Since men tend to be bottom-line-oriented, the easy-to-discern advantages of cosmetic surgery are quite persuasive.

VIVE LA DIFFÉRENCE!

If men and women are different on so many fronts—from biology to brain chemistry—then it makes sense that our skin differs, too. Male skin tends to be thicker and remain elastic longer. Men wrinkle less because they have more collagen, a protein responsible for the plumpness beneath the skin. Also in men, fat under the skin tends to be firmer and more vascular, so many of the newest liposuction techniques, such as ultrasound assisted lipoplasty (UAL) and power assisted lipoplasty (PAL), in which fat is broken up before it is removed, are especially effective. There are other physical differences that make for a cosmetic surgery gender gap. Muscles are thicker in men. Male facial skin has a richer blood supply due to facial hair; thus men tend to bleed more during surgery, and have a greater tendency (though still small) to get post-operative hematomas. Men also typically require more anesthesia.

As for aesthetics, it's harder for men to hide scars, because generally they don't have available to them the concealing agents that women do—makeup and longer, fuller hair. Of course, beards, mustaches, and full sideburns help obscure facial scarring in a way unavailable to women. Make sure you discuss with your surgeon where he or she plans to make incisions, so that you are comfortable with their size, number, and placement. Finally, we assess proportion differently when working on a man's face. For example, a male face with a weak chin suffers much more then a female one. And since lines, and even scars, on a man's face are often considered macho, rugged, or sexy, a more limited procedure might still yield a very nice result.

The distinctive psychology of men may be the biggest challenge for surgeons. Men tend to approach surgery with a very different outlook from that of women. For the most part, men want to come in, have the thing done, and get out. While most of my female patients and I have developed close relationships, it's not always so with my male patients, even my repeaters. Many of them treat their surgeon much the way they might treat their interior decorator: "Here's what I want, now do it, and don't tell me the details." Recently, a high-level financial executive came in wanting to have his eyes done. I sat down, ready to talk about what was involved and the various choices he had to consider. "I don't want to discuss it," he said. "Whatever you need to do, do!" Since my approach is *It's your body; I give you the options; you make the final decision*, I practically had to force him to listen to the choices before him. Ultimately, I recommended an endoscopic forehead lift, and not surprisingly, he agreed. I think that many men feel that laying it all out—the initial desire to have the cosmetic surgery, the choices, the details, the implications—amplifies the vanity of the procedure. It's more difficult for them to say exactly what bothers them or how much, whereas women know their faces intimately and have no trouble discussing how they feel about this line or that spot. This makes for a paradox in men's behavior: On the one hand, they can be direct and unambiguous; on the other, they can be vague and unnervingly acquiescent.

In practical terms, the male perspective can cause post-operative problems. Since men tend not to ask for help during recovery, they may get depressed. They also tend to be impatient. Many men don't like to rest, and their activity can lead to post-operative bleeding and infection. Some even want to drive themselves home after surgery. As a group, men are often accused of having a lower threshold for pain than women, but I find this is largely dependent on the individual, the surgery involved, and other circumstances.

In their defense, men are simply not used to all the fixings and trimmings and buffings that women are from their visits to the beauty salon and manicurist, and so physical prodding and scrutiny of their features make them uncomfortable. As a result, I need to be clever about getting men to follow instructions. For instance, when I recommend a skin-care regimen for a man, I might start him with a single product, not the several I tend to recommend for women. My goal is to get him to see results with the first product. Only then can I recommend more and know that he's willing to follow the plan, morning and night.

Virtually all the procedures favored by my male patients are explained in detail in earlier chapters, so I'll focus here on the special considerations associated with each of the top ten surgeries requested by men.

LIPOSUCTION

Nine times out of ten I use liposuction, not a lift or tuck, to resculpt a man's body. One reason is that men's skin tends to contract especially well after lipo. Another—and let's be honest here—is that we don't hold men to the same high aesthetic standards to which we hold women. So what if they have a little wrinkle here or there, or a lumpy patch of skin? Flaws and sags that might be obvious in a woman are easily camouflaged by a man's facial or body hair.

Since weight accumulates differently in men than in women, the sources of greatest concern and dismay differ, too. The most popular areas for male liposuction are the waist ("love handles"), abdomen (potbelly), chest, and neck. To reduce love handles or a "beer gut," a tiny incision is made in the navel and the fat is suctioned out with a cannula, a small probing tube attached to a vacuum; to get rid of a jowly neck, the incision is placed discreetly right beneath the chin.

Men are an easy sell when it comes to liposuction. Jim, a computer executive in his forties, first came to see me for an eyelid lift to open his drooping lids. Six months later he was back for lipo on his stomach, breasts, and neck. "It would never have occurred to me to go in for another procedure," says Jim, "but in the follow-up visits for my eyes I got comfortable with the idea, and I found I could break through some of my mental barriers regarding cosmetic surgery. The doctor told me that the next thing she was thinking about fixing was my neck, which was gaining some heft. I said that actually I'd been thinking about my stomach, since over the previous few years I'd felt as if I'd been carrying around an additional ten to fifteen pounds in the form of a little bowling ball." We did both procedures, and I know Jim was happy he went for the whole thing. "I could see the difference the next day," he says. "I have a twenty-two-year-old son, and we play a lot of sports together. I no longer feel as if I've got that extra weight holding me back. I also think the surgery was good for my career. When you get a little older, the weight can give you the appearance of laziness. I think looking fitter projects a higher degree of productivity."

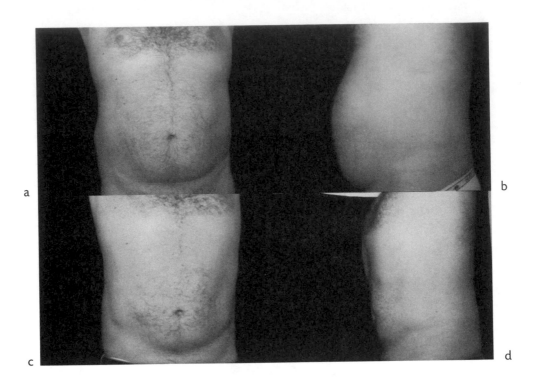

a

b

c

d

ABDOMINAL LIPOSUCTION

Men are more likely than women to get potbellies, even when they exercise (a, b). This is easily fixed through liposuction performed through a tiny hole in the navel, as was done on this thirty-nine-year-old accountant (c, d). While he'll need to watch his weight, one thing is for sure: The fat will never gather in the same spot again.

Liposuction, with its circumscribed recovery period (surgery is typically followed by three to seven days of bruising, tenderness, and/or numbness around the incision sites, though patients can return to work after only a couple of days), is a quick, relatively painless way of resculpting the body.

ABDOMINOPLASTY (TUMMY TUCK)

I seldom do this procedure on male patients, because men rarely suffer from excessively hanging abdominal skin. For men with good skin elasticity, liposuction is just as effective at getting rid of a potbelly that hasn't responded to diet and exercise. With lipo, the procedure can be done in an hour through a tiny hole in the navel, while a tummy tuck is a lengthy, riskier procedure that leaves the patient with a hip-to-hip scar. I make an exception for men with hanging skin in the midriff area due to massive weight loss or very loose muscles. The procedure removes excess fat, tightens the muscles of the abdominal wall, and trims the waistline. The recovery for this surgery is notably long: Often, you can't return to work for at least two weeks after the operation while the tissues are healing.

FACE-LIFT/MINI-LIFT

The nipping and tucking that an older face may require is roughly the same whether that face belongs to a woman or a man; indeed, I see lots of couples come in—wives dragging husbands, girlfriends with boyfriends—wanting me to do the identical procedure on both. As explained in Chapter 8, I prefer a mini-lift in conjuction with an endoscopic forehead lift, to achieve the results of a full face-lift. There's far less scarring and less downtime, and the results are more natural than after a traditional face-lift. A mini-lift eliminates jowls and loose skin in the lower face, and the particulars for a male and female patient are the same, with one exception: On a woman, I start the incision at the top of the ear and take it behind the tragus (the bump at the front of the ear) to maximally hide the scar. In a man, the incision runs from the top of the ear *in front* of the tragus. For both men and women, the incision continues under the lobe and into the natural fold where the earlobe meets the cheek. Making the incision in front of the tragus prevents an embarrassing scenario: having whisker-growing skin literally pulled into the ear. (The whisker hairline along the jaw may also be pulled back *behind* the ear, creating the ridiculous predicament of having to shave there. If this somehow happens, don't panic: Laser treatment eliminates hair growth in awkward places.)

The procedure takes a couple of hours and has a downtime of about two weeks. You'll most likely have bruising and swelling around the lower face and neck, but as long as you follow your doctor's instructions, keep your head elevated, and ice the affected areas, you should feel and look much better in just a few days.

If you have deep facial creasing and other signs of aging above the nose, the mini-lift may not do as much as you'd like, and an endoscopic forehead lift may be a better option.

ENDOSOCOPIC FOREHEAD LIFT

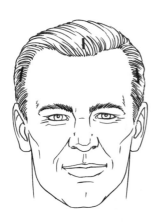

MALE ENDOSCOPIC
FOREHEAD LIFT
INCISION SITES

The traditional, big-incision forehead lift was, for a long time, a no-no for the follically challenged man whose receding hairline would reveal every inch of the scar. But now that we've perfected the endoscopic, small-incision forehead lift, even bald men can enjoy great results. The surgeon makes quarter-inch incisions on top of the head (see illustration) and inserts an endoscope—a tube-shaped probe with a camera on one end—to see what's going on underneath the skin. He or she then separates the underlying tissue, muscle, and skin from the bone and lifts everything to smooth out the saggy brow and deep forehead wrinkles. The skin is then sutured in its new, higher position. (If the patient is not yet bald, but clearly exhibits male-pattern baldness, the surgeon should factor that in when making incisions, anticipating that in several years the scars will not be concealed the way they are now.)

This remarkably quick procedure takes about one hour. You can expect bruising and temporary numbness around the eyes and midface, but most of my patients report that the recovery isn't painful, just uncomfortable.

NECK LIPECTOMY

If all I need to do to a face is eliminate jowls and neck bulge, then a neck lipectomy often suffices. In younger patients, a doughy double chin can easily be suctioned out in a matter of minutes through lipo. However, older patients

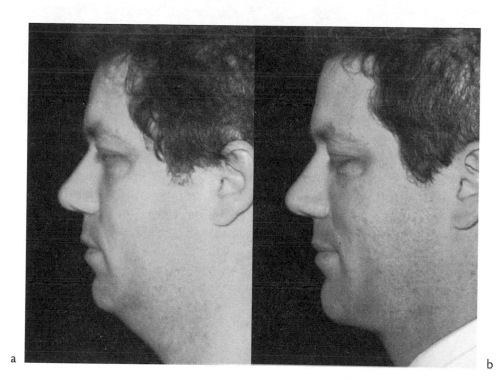

a

b

NECK LIPECTOMY WITH CHIN IMPLANT

Nothing adds years and pounds to a person's appearance like a pudgy, droopy neck (a). I performed a neck lipectomy on this forty-seven-year-old attorney, sucking out fat and tightening the neck muscles through a small hole under the chin. I also decided to give him a chin implant to more clearly define his neckline. He had the procedure on a Thursday and was back at work the next Monday, looking like a new man (b).

and those who suffer from a loose "gobble neck" may require a neck lift that includes the removal of excess skin and tightening of the platysma muscles, which run down the front of the neck. The procedure can last one to two hours, and usually results in temporary bruising and soreness around the neck and collarbone area. Because gravity pulls the bruising downward, you may be able to return to work after only a few days, as a shirt can hide any telltale black-and-blue marks (but don't cinch your tie too tight!). For best results, this procedure may be performed in conjunction with chin augmentation.

CHIN AUGMENTATION

A man can hide a weak chin behind his beard. But why resort to such elaborate grooming when the problem can be so easily fixed? For this procedure, which takes roughly an hour to perform, the surgeon makes a small incision under the chin and inserts the implant through it. Male chin implants tend to be larger than women's, because the male face proportionally can support a stronger chin; in fact, the chin is even something of a "statement" feature on a man, a sign of strong character. "My receding chin seemed wimpy," says Sheldon, a sixty-eight-year-old retired sales executive. After a chin implant and necklift to eliminate his wattly chin, Sheldon reports, "I feel more assertive and commanding."

Post-operative bruising in the chin and neck areas is easily concealed by a beard (shaving one's beard is not required before this operation). Be careful when shaving, however, to avoid nicking yourself at the incision site.

EYELID LIFT (BLEPHAROPLASTY)

Puffy eyes or droopy lids make a man look tired and older than his years, and he can't resort to a woman's trick of using liner and mascara to give his eyes more definition. A blepharoplasty or eyelid lift, in which fatty tissue underneath the upper and lower lids is excised (or redistributed) and excess skin removed, can "open" and brighten the eyes. The incision along the upper crease and lower lashes will be virtually invisible when it heals. If there is puffiness around the eyes but minimal droop, a surgeon should arguably cut out the excess from inside the lids so there is no visible scarring, as is often done for women. The procedure takes about an hour, and, though you'll need someone to take you home and periodically assist you in putting ointment in your eyes (your vision may be blurred upon waking from surgery), the healing time for blepharoplasty is a relatively quick four to five days.

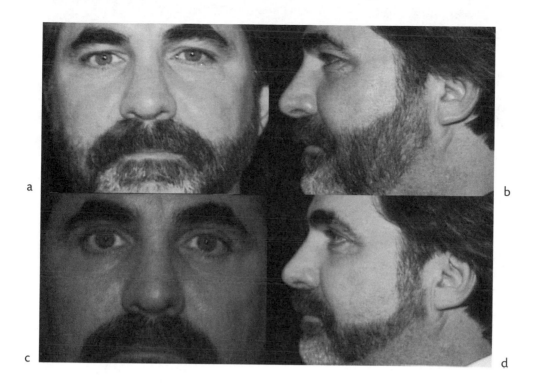

a   b   c   d

EYELID LIFT

When everyone at work kept teasing him about about how tired he looked, this forty-five-year-old computer executive came to see me about improving his droopy lids and dark circles (a, b). I started him on a skin-care regimen to help lighten the tissue around the eyes, then performed an upper and lower blepharoplasty to remove excess tissue and fat. His eyes look as they must have more than ten years ago (c, d).

MALE BREAST REDUCTION

Many men, including teens, are too ashamed of their overdeveloped breasts to take off their shirt at the beach. The common condition known as *gynecomastia* (Greek for "womanlike breasts") is characterized by enlarged breast tissue. We're not sure what causes it; gynecomastia seems to have no connection to obesity, and it often, though not always, begins during puberty. The origin can be genetic, hormonal, a medical condition like an impaired liver or testicular tumor, or the result of the use or abuse of substances like anabolic steroids,

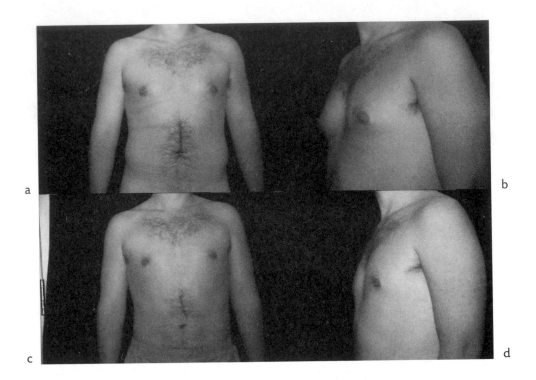

a

b

c

d

SURGERY FOR GYNECOMASTIA

Although this patient wasn't overweight, he collected fat in his love handles and suffered from gynecomastia, the enlargement of the male breast (a, b). When he was thirty-two and could finally afford surgery, he came to me for liposuction on his hips and breasts. The scars, which are on his back and just under the nipple, are almost invisible (c, d).

---

estrogen-containing medications, marijuana, or alcohol. It may occur in both breasts or one. Gynecomastia affects an astonishing 40 to 60 percent of men, and, when extreme, can be emotionally and socially devastating. Recalls George, a twenty-six-year-old media planner:

"Ever since puberty I'd had enlarged breasts. I dreaded putting myself in any situation where I'd have to take off my shirt, like the locker room or the beach. I would actually swim in a shirt! And dating? Forget it. I was way too embarrassed to ever let a woman see me without clothes. It got to the point where I

felt I was really missing out on a normal life, but I worked out constantly and could never do anything to diminish the problem. I had no idea there was something surgical I could do about it."

Fortunately, the condition is easily reversed with liposuction. The surgeon will make a small incision, three to four millimeters long, under the nipple, at the edge of the areola (some doctors make their incision in the underarm). I tend to use a type of liposuction that involves ultrasound to liquefy the fat to make its removal easier. Whatever the method used, the surgeon will eventually suck out the fat and glandular tissue from around the areola and from the sides and bottom of the breasts. With overweight men the process is tougher, because they may have sagging skin that needs to be tucked. The incisions are covered with dressings, and the patient has to wear a compression garment around his torso for a week to ten days to help keep the repositioned skin firmly in place.

This surgery is not recommended for children or most teens, since the problem will likely resolve itself: 90 percent of cases disappear within two years of their onset. There are exceptions for some teens who suffer greatly from the shattered self-confidence of enduring such a condition when body image is so dominant a concern. If the condition appears in adulthood, it may be caused by drug or steroid abuse—especially among avid weightlifters. In an attempt to reduce the obviousness of their condition, some men bulk up, though in fact this will probably only worsen it.

The procedure generally takes one-and-a-half to two hours. It's not necessary to trim or shave chest hair beforehand; in fact, the hair will help camouflage the scars as they heal. This surgery is sometimes covered by insurance, and is more likely to be covered for a teen suffering from the condition.

Problems one may experience after this surgery include skin loss at the incision sites, permanent pigment changes in the breast area, and slightly mismatched breasts or nipples, which can be easily fixed through a second procedure. Another possible complication is "saucer deformity," a craterlike irregularity that can result from poor liposuction technique or poor healing ability. There's also the potential for numbness or loss of sensation in the breast for up to a year.

LASER HAIR REMOVAL

An excessively hairy chest wasn't always considered unappealing. But in recent years, the "clean" look of a hairless chest has grown in popularity, and a more-than-modest amount of hair is often considered a turn-off. Fortunately, a new generation of lasers has been developed for more effective hair removal, especially for those who want to eliminate hair on the back, shoulders, and chest. How does it work? The laser energy deactivates hair follicles and stops hair from growing. However, since it grows at different rates, not all the offending hair is eliminated with one treatment. (Women who wax already know this.) As a result, you may need multiple treatments—sometimes up to four or five, depending on the type of laser and body part. The only side effects are a temporary burning sensation and slight skin irritation. Laser hair removal also helps prevent the common and annoying problem of ingrown hairs (*folliculitis*) caused by shaving and waxing. For that reason alone, many men find this new laser technology to be a great option.

OTHER QUICK FIXES

Hair removal is just one of the most popular laser treatments for men. I use lasers—as well as resurfacing procedures such as microdermabrasion—with increasing frequency on my male patients, who now come seeking to rid themselves of cosmetic distractions as often as they come seeking surgical rejuvenation of the face and body. We also use lasers to minimize acne scarring, diminish age spots, remove spider veins, and tighten loose or jowly skin. (For more information on these techniques, see Chapters 6 and 7.)

MUSCLE ENHANCEMENT

While proving effective in many cases so far, muscle enhancement surgery is still relatively new, and it's not that easy to find someone qualified to perform this type of procedure.

The idea of muscle enhancement is to improve contour through cosmetic implants and sculpting techniques. Calf implants, for example, create fullness in the lower leg; pectoral implants help to bulk the look of the pec muscles ("chest buffing"). Some doctors also offer male patients "abdominal etching," a new liposuction technique that results in a highly muscular, "ripped" appearance in the stomach.

Besides the lack of well-trained surgeons to perform these operations, there's another problem: Synthetic material is typically used in these implants, and that may not be ideal. It may move if jostled, and scar tissue can ultimately form around an implant, causing stiffness and/or pain and limited mobility.

FIGHTING AGE IN A JAR

I never look to solve a problem surgically if an easier, less expensive, equally effective solution is available. That's why I encourage men to follow a skin-care regimen to help prevent the visible signs of aging that cause even the toughest of guys to look in the mirror with dismay. There are now many over-the-counter cosmetics lines aimed at men. Pick one that includes glycolic acids, which exfoliate the top layer of skin and stimulate regeneration in a gentle way, and an antioxidant like vitamin C, which battles damaging free radicals and increases skin elasticity. A daily moisturizer will help keep skin cells moist and plump. (Like many dermatologists and plastic surgeons, I have tailored a skin-care program specifically for men. For information, see www.drmichellecopelandskincare.com.) Finally, don't forget to wear sunscreen regularly—even on those spur-of-the-moment runs or golf outings. Nothing ages the skin faster than the sun's ultraviolet light (to say nothing of the higher probability of developing skin cancer with prolonged sun exposure). And no: A baseball cap isn't sufficient protection.

Countless men have now learned that cosmetic enhancement isn't about vanity, but about taking a constructive approach to solving a physical problem with emotional resonance. Just as for women, finding a surgical solution to a long-term problem improves men's looks *and* their lives. And, as has been my experience with so many male patients, it frequently triggers a broader commitment to healthier habits.

12

Healing: Making It Quicker and Easier

Surgery is only the midway point in the overall care I give my patients. To me, being a plastic surgeon isn't just doing what we do in the operating room. It includes weeks, even months, of follow-ups to monitor the healing process and to make sure patients' recoveries are healthy, happy, and as easy and stress-free as possible.

I advocate a holistic approach, taking into account both a patient's physical and emotional well-being. I use massage therapy, customized exercise programs, and a wide variety of healing methods to reduce swelling and bruising, and to make sure that the patient enjoys a speedy recovery.

THE HEALING BEGINS *BEFORE* SURGERY

Healing is not an exclusively post-surgery process. If you prepare adequately for surgery, you will sow the seeds for a quicker, easier, less painful recovery afterward.

Pre-Op Guidelines

As a patient, there are many things that you should do in the weeks and days leading to surgery, including several that directly involve your surgeon. Make sure that your prospective doctor (or nurse):

◆ administers to you any necessary pre-operative tests, such as a physical, blood work, or an EKG, depending on your age;

◆ has taken a "before" photograph of you for reference during surgery;

◆ has explained in detail your procedure, where your incisions will be located, what recovery entails, and the protocol for post-surgical follow-up.

This is the checklist I give my patients:

✔ Two weeks prior to surgery, take a multivitamin once a day to boost your nutritional status in preparation for the recovery, when the body will crave replenishment. (If you already take a multi, continue your regimen.)

✔ **Avoid the following medications and supplements within two weeks of the operation to aid clotting and minimize bruising:**

 • aspirin or aspirin-containing products (a single aspirin before surgery can impair the platelet function necessary for blood clotting);

 • anti-inflammatory medications like ibuprofen (found in OTCs like Advil and Motrin);

 • Vitamin E or Vitamin E–containing products (a blood thinner, E is found in many "health-food" shakes and energy bars);

 • antihistamines in cold and allergy pills;

 • guaifenesin (found in some cough syrups and cold medications);

 • some herbs and herbal supplements, including willow bark (whose active ingredient, salicin, is a precursor of aspirin), digitalis (a source of some cardiac medicines), echinacea (reputed to cause blood pressure abnormalities when used with anesthesia), ginkgo biloba (which has an anticoagulant effect), and pineapple extract (which some claim reduces swelling).

✔ *Tell your doctor if you're on any medication, including statins, hormones, or antidepressants.* Some of these medications may interfere with healing, or may produce a negative reaction when taken in conjunction with other drugs connected with surgery. Do not be embarrassed to tell your doctor what you are taking (Viagra, for instance)—it is vital for your health that we know.

✔ If you get cold sores, tell your doctor too—they are triggered by stress and may interfere with healing from facial surgery.

✔ Fill prescriptions for any post-operative medications your surgeon has required *before* surgery.

✔ Line up a trusted person to accompany you home from the doctor's office. You'll most likely be on bed rest for at least the first twenty-four hours. Depending on the type of surgery, you may want someone to stay with you during your first night.

✔ Set up your home so that amenities (compress, water, tissues, etc.) are bedside, and keep clutter minimal.

✔ For face-lift/brow lift candidates: If you color your hair, have it done as close as possible to the surgery date. You won't be able to use hair dyes again for at least one month.

✔ Choose a comfortable outfit for the day of surgery that may be put on easily after the procedure. For face, neck, or breast surgery, avoid wearing shirts or sweaters that you'll have to pull over your head. For certain skin procedures, such as laser resurfacing or glycolic peels, bring a large scarf to conceal any resulting redness or discoloration on the trip home.

✔ Don't eat or drink after midnight the night before surgery.

✔ Avoid spicy foods (such as Thai or Chinese) for a full day before surgery. Salt, spices, and other seasonings promote inflammation.

✔ Avoid alcohol the day before surgery for the same reason.

✔ Shower the night before or morning of surgery, because you won't be able to do it again for at least two days post-op. Don't apply perfume, deodorant, or other chemicals near the surgical site; doing so risks infection.

✔ Don't wear makeup to your surgery. Keep your face and hands clean.

✔ For face-lifts and eye surgery, don't wear contact lenses (and prepare to possibly go without glasses for some time after the procedure).

(PLASTIC) SURGEON'S GENERAL WARNING: STOP SMOKING!

Smoking triggers the release of skin-damaging free radicals, increases swelling, worsens scarring, and impedes healing by limiting blood flow to the skin. If you smoke, you should refrain for at least two weeks before your procedure and two weeks after. That's a month without nicotine, during a time when you're likely to be anxious about undergoing and recovering from surgery. Since cutting out cigarettes will undoubtedly frazzle you further, I'd far prefer it, of course, if you started cutting back well before that two-week sentence. (Read my lips: Quit.) But given the difficulty of what I'm asking, try a prescription or over-the-counter anti-smoking product to help you bridge the time until you can once again light up, if you must. Among the other threats that smoking poses is the distinct chance that you won't be able to find a self-respecting surgeon to perform the desired procedure. Wouldn't this be the perfect occasion to seriously try to kick the habit?

PARTNERS IN RECOVERY

No matter how big or small the procedure, surgery is a stressful experience. Patients worry about the pain, what they're going to look like afterward, how they'll manage their time away from the office and a reduced exercise schedule. Since stress hormones can hamper the healing process, it is especially important for doctors to help patients come out of surgery in the right frame of mind.

Most surgeons, myself included, give patients a list of post-op do's and don'ts about taking pain medication and avoiding infection, and self-care recommendations for bathing, eating, sleeping, and exercising. This list shouldn't feel Draconian—patients have a life they need to resume. In fact, a forward-thinking doctor will urge a high degree of pro-activity for his or her patients, encouraging them to feel empowered to take charge of their own healing. As a patient in recovery, you need to listen to your body and judge what you can and can't physically accomplish. Restrictions on your mobility needn't be life-stopping.

And for all the careful work that a surgeon does, both in the operating room and afterward, *you're* the one responsible for your own recovery. Although your doctor can monitor you in follow-up visits and over the phone, he or she can't be there every step of the way. The healing process is collaborative, and you need to hold up your end of the bargain.

HOW WE HEAL

A Scar Is Born

There's no such thing as surgery without a scar (doctors who tell you otherwise are lying). There are some procedures, such as liposuction and breast implantation, that give us a choice about where to place the scar and how big or visible it will be. Fortunately, for all procedures, we now have several ways to minimize the amount of noticeable scarring with which you'll be left.

Healing begins right after an incision is made. Cells and natural chemical substances rush to the affected area, causing edema (swelling). After a few days, cells called fibroblasts begin to produce the protein collagen, which is found in all skin and is the main component of scar tissue. The body, in effect, is sealing itself from outside infection. But sometimes collagen can overreact, resulting in raised, red scars called keloids. Some people are genetically programmed to respond with this kind of scarring; you probably know from getting other cuts and scrapes over the years if you're one of them. What's more, because collagen is produced in different amounts all over the body, not all body parts heal at the same rate, or with the same degree of smoothness (the neck and hands, for instance, are particularly prone to scar formation, while the face and torso tend to scar less easily).

There are several steps you can take to minimize scarring. If you start treatment early, topical steroids can help diminish scar formation by changing the configuration of the collagen (meaning that the fibers that make up collagen are softened). A steroid can also be injected directly into a keloid to soften it. Silicone-based creams and gels, when applied directly to the scar, effectively smooth its texture. I start my patients on all three regimens as soon as the incision has healed (usually two to three weeks after surgery).

The healing process should be hands-on. I've found that through massage therapy I can manually mold scars as they form. Gentle massage directly on and around a scar in a small circular motion, starting two to three weeks after surgery, can make the new collagen softer and suppler, as it is essentially breaking down the bands of tissue. Massage can also help return sensation to the area around the incision, which can be numb for several days or weeks, by stimulating the ingrowth of new nerve endings. (However, don't massage your scar without your doctor's consent.)

Scars also have a tendency to become discolored. Traumatized skin responds in one of two ways: It can form too little pigment or too much. If you even out the pigment formation as it occurs, the scar will be neither too light nor too dark. To do that, you can apply a pigment blocking cream to inhibit the production of melanin, the substance responsible for skin color (paradoxically, it works on people who produce too little pigment as well as those who produce too much). The most effective products contain hydroquinone or kojic acid. Thyme—yes, the herb, which is an ingredient in some skin creams—also functions as a pigment blocker, but isn't as potent as the chemical products. If discoloration persists, a laser can be used to make the pigment more uniform.

Finally, some routine methods we use on the skin help minimize the appearance of scars and promote an overall healthy look. Exfoliating with light glycolic acids stimulates cell turnover, forcing the skin to regenerate and heal. Wearing moisturizing cream helps mend skin that has been stressed and traumatized. I put all my patients, who've had everything from lipo to breast surgery, on a rigorous skin-care program starting days after their surgery to help the skin contract and heal. The regimen includes showering with a gentle cleanser, exfoliating, and moisturizing.

URGENT QUESTION:
HOW CAN I TELL IF MY SCAR IS INFECTED?

In the two- to three-week period when a scar is forming, it will look red and puffy. Some swelling is natural, and you can manage it by applying a cold compress to the area for twenty minutes a couple of times a day. But when the swelling becomes fiery or pulls at the sutures, that's a sign of infection. Fever is another sign.

Infection can set in as a result of clothing rubbing on the incision, which opens the scab and makes way for bacteria; it may also happen if you sweat near the incision site or touch the area with dirty hands. Your surgeon will show you how to keep your scar clean. You will probably have to wear a surgical dressing for the first twenty-four to seventy-two hours after your procedure. Once the dressing is removed, keep the wound clean with hydrogen peroxide and a topical antibiotic. If you get an infection, contact your doctor immediately.

You won't know for some time how your scar will ultimately look. A scar can be most noticeable at six weeks, when it will appear red and puffy. This is when collagen production has reached its height. But a scar can take up to a year to finish forming. Occasionally, a patient will come to me before then, unhappy with the way his or her scar looks. In rare cases, as I mentioned earlier, a scar can grow a keloid, assuming a dark red, ropy quality. After a couple of months we can consider a high-tech scar-smoothing procedure, such as microdermabrasion or laser treatment. To perform a scar revision—where a scar is excised and the area resutured—we would have to wait several more months, and this is something that usually can be avoided by the interventions described above.

NEW SCAR FIXERS

In lieu of traditional sutures, some surgeons are using newly developed glues to close up incisions, and tissue sealants created from fibrin (a substance the body makes naturally in scar formation) to help tissues adhere. These hold promise for the future, but I don't think there's enough research yet to warrant their use. The procedures can be cumbersome and costly, and they add a new risk of infection. Is it worth the gamble, just to get around the (admittedly) exacting process of making a few stitches in the skin? I, for one, don't think so—at least right now.

Looking (and Feeling) Blue

Some people are especially prone to bruising and emerge from surgery looking like they've just been through several rounds with Mike Tyson. Others have no trace of black or blue even a couple of days post-op.

Bruising is caused by local bleeding or the pooling of blood beneath the skin. It's a far more common occurrence with general anesthesia than with local, because local anesthetics contain epinephrine, a naturally occurring chemical that causes the veins to constrict, minimizing blood loss. New instruments are also less traumatic to body tissues, reducing the chance of bruising; the Ultrasound Assisted Lipoplasty (UAL) instrument, for instance, uses radio frequency waves to break up the fat underneath the skin, making its removal easier. And the cannulas now used for traditional liposuction are much narrower. The tight garments that lipo patients have to wear for the first week or so also reduce bruising by restricting fluid accumulation.

Certain drugs and supplements impede clotting and increase the risk of bruising, and should be avoided *before* surgery (see the list on pages 230–231). Some patients ask me whether arnica decreases bruising, but I don't recommend it as it is an uncontrolled substance and may cause an adverse reaction.

Most bruising should disappear within two to three weeks, and some patients heal even faster. In the meantime, there are several steps you can take to conceal your blemishes: Wear special camouflaging makeup containing pigments that neutralize blue and yellow; keep your hair down to cover facial or neck bruises; or wear clothes that cover the affected area without constricting it.

TAKING CHARGE OF YOUR RECOVERY

When something goes wrong in the healing process, it's usually because a patient is bucking his or her doctor's guidelines. The person may do so out of laziness, but more likely it's out of cockiness, or an underestimation of what it takes for the body to repair itself. I once had a patient who felt so good within a few days of having a tummy tuck that she went dancing—and promptly tore her incision. A rhinoplasty patient wore his nose splint into the shower the day of his operation, and the splint slid off. Yet another patient couldn't stay off the phone after a face-lift and developed an infection near her ear. Make sure you don't become one of these unfortunate few. Adhere to your doctor's recommendations and arm yourself with the knowledge of how to help your body heal.

Getting Comfortable at Home

◆ **Recruit help.** You will be on bed rest for at least the first twenty-four hours and will need to arrange for someone to stay with you during that time. Some may find comfort in a helping hand, but others, used to living alone or wanting to hide their condition from the outside world, may feel it an imposition. Believe me: You cannot, and should not, go it alone. Even if your procedure is done under twilight sedation, rather than general anesthesia, it may take a few hours to feel fully alert. After many types of surgery (including breast surgery, tummy tucks, and liposuction), you are forbidden from lifting *any* weight, so even carrying a pitcher of water or taking down a blanket from a closet is out of the question. If you don't have a family member or friend who can pitch in, your doctor can help arrange for a visiting nurse, which can run from $20 to $75 per hour.

◆ **Prep your pad.** Don't leave yourself, or your helper, with too much to do when you return from the doctor. It's smart to equip your recovery room—be it a bedroom, den, or hotel room—with a post-surgery kit in advance. This kit should include:

- A copy of your doctor's post-op instructions.

- Tylenol or another medication for pain, fever, and swelling (consult your doctor about which).

- Bendable straws for sipping liquid, if you are having a face-lift, necklift, or rhinoplasty.

- Ice packs. Many patients find that bags of frozen peas are ideal, since they mold to the body nicely and won't melt all over you. A less pungent option: gel packs that can be refrozen.

- Two large clean towels. Put these over your pillowcase to help keep your sheets clean as the wound heals.

- Two to three large pillows.

◆ **Limit visitors.** Not that you'll want your office mates and book-club friends to see you in all your post-operative glory, but even well-wishing family members should be discouraged from visiting during the first couple of days. The body heals more quickly when it is resting, and a steady stream of visitors can wear you out. The last thing you need is to be jumping up and down offering guests drinks and snacks.

◆ **Chill out.** You may have been saving *War and Peace* for a rainy day, but don't count on getting past the first chapter. If you've had facial surgery—especially an eyelid lift or rhinoplasty—you may find wearing glasses uncomfortable for a couple of weeks, and contacts are forbidden. So books and even TV may be out of the question, as well as bill-paying and desk work. If you must seek distraction, stock up on music CDs and books on tape. And opt for e-mail over phone use: Facial surgery patients won't be able to hold a phone to their ear for the first week or two.

◆ **Eating and drinking.** On your first night at home, you can have water, ice chips, juice, or caffeine-free soda. Avoid alcohol, which can interfere with your medication, and caffeinated drinks, which can disrupt sleep. Drink enough liquids: The body needs ample water for cells to mend. Depending on the type of surgery you've had (this is particularly true for abdominal surgery), you may also want to limit your food intake to soft fare such as Jell-O, scrambled eggs, or yogurt.

◆ **Ice, ice, ice.** An ice pack greatly reduces swelling (those gel packs or bags of frozen peas are ideal, because they mold to the body). Never place ice directly on the skin; rather, be sure to wrap a cloth around it to dull the chill. Most doctors recommend icing for twenty minutes, with a twenty-minute break, on and off for the first twenty-four hours.

◆ **Keep your dressing clean.** After nearly all surgeries, a sterile dressing—anything from small adhesive bandages to gauze wrappings—is placed over the incisions to maintain a clean environment and prevent infection. These usually stay on for up to a week. Depending on the surgery, you may have to return to the doctor a day or two later to have your dressing changed. If you need to do it yourself (if you live too far away for a return visit), get careful instructions from your doctor.

◆ **Medication.** Follow your doctor's instructions regarding pain relievers and antibiotics, and check with him or her before taking any over-the-counter painkillers, especially aspirin or ibuprofen, which can affect blood clotting.

◆ **Elevation.** Almost all patients can expect some swelling after surgery. Keeping the affected areas of the body elevated for the first two days will help minimize swelling and prevent edema (excessive fluid accumulation). If surgery was performed on the face, neck, or breasts, you'll need to lie or sit with your head propped up on a couple of pillows. Two or three pillows under the legs and/or midsection offer sufficient elevation after liposuction or a tummy tuck.

◆ **Sleeping.** Most patients find it difficult to sleep after cosmetic surgery. For the first few days, you'll need to sleep in the same elevated position that you maintain during the day. If you've had surgery on the upper body, you may find it more comfortable to sleep in a recliner than a bed. Sleep is an important part of the healing process, as the body shifts into repair mode when its other faculties shut down. If you have trouble falling asleep, try a cup of chamomile tea or warm milk. I don't advocate sleeping pills, because being truly conked out limits your movement during sleep, and movement is necessary to help prevent edema (the exception is abdominal surgery, after which you should keep your torso as still as possible for the first twenty-four hours). And limit your intake of caffeine, especially before bed.

◆ **Bathing and hygiene.** So long as the sutures are visible, avoid their immersion in water. I use dissolving sutures for nearly all the procedures I perform, but there are many surgeons who still use traditional sutures or staples, which need to be removed after seven days. A warm sponge bath is an easy solution. Have a friend or family member help you, if necessary. Once the sutures come out or dissolve, it's okay to take a shower, though you should avoid total immersion for two weeks.

◆ **Movement and exercise.** I once had a liposuction patient who was so afraid that movement would tug at her incisions that she stayed absolutely still for nearly two days. Her legs swelled up like torpedoes, because gravity caused the blood to pool in her lower extremities. Not only does being sedentary slow the recovery process, it can be dangerous. Lots of evidence suggests that moderate movement is beneficial for healing. It constricts blood vessels after surgery, reducing the amount of substances in the bloodstream that cause swelling. In some cases, movement actually helps tissue mend. With breast augmentation, for instance, upper-body exercise (such as light weight training) can reduce capsular contracture, the formation of scar tissue around the implants. If you feel up to it a day or two after surgery, go for an easy walk. Just don't raise your blood pressure too high while healing, which may result in bleeding. As long as you continue to wear a surgical dressing or a compression garment, you should not break a sweat, which can lead to infection. After two weeks or so, you can increase the intensity of your workout a notch (see guidelines on exercise, pages 244–245, increasing gradually after the wound heals completely.

The Healing Powers of Massage

One week after their procedure, I have most patients come in for a post-surgical lymphatic massage. This is a light-touch massage given by a trained therapist, which stimulates the lymph system, ridding it of impurities and chemicals that cause and prolong swelling. Because the surgery site is still healing, the therapist touches only near sites on the face, scalp, and neck, where the lymph nodes drain.

Perhaps almost more important, massage is a relaxant. Massage therapy has been shown to short-circuit the body's stress response (known also as the "fight or flight" impulse) by boosting the production of endorphins, the body's feel-good hormones, and reducing the level of sympathetic hormones, such as adrenaline, that cause the pulse to race. Relaxing the body creates an environment conducive to healing. If your surgeon doesn't offer massage at your follow-up appointments, book your own in consultation with the doctor.

NEW ALTERNATIVES

I've found lymphatic massage to be crucial to recovery. Other alternative therapies that help patients relax and promote healing include acupuncture, reflexology, hypnosis, and Reiki therapy (an energy manipulation technique). I can't offer scientific proof that they have a direct effect on pain or on the healing of tissues, per se. But I've seen that they make patients feel good, and I'm willing to incorporate whatever makes the surgical and post-surgical experience less stressful to my patients.

Guidelines to Observe in the Coming Weeks

◆ **Returning to work.** When you go back to the office depends, of course, on the kind of surgery you've had and your body's response to it. Liposuction typically requires very little downtime because the incisions are tiny, and patients can wear body-concealing clothes. I've even known patients who have gone out to dinner a couple of days after a rhinoplasty, flaunting their splint for all to see. More commonly, though, especially after facial surgery, patients want to stay out of public scrutiny for at least a week until their bruises heal, the swelling begins to subside, and they feel stronger and ready to confront the world. Although we now have many procedures that allow you to be up and about almost immediately, there's a danger in doing too much too soon. A breast implant patient who totes a heavy briefcase to and from work puts stress on her sutures. A patient who has had liposuction on his stomach and sits all day at his desk risks having his skin adhere unevenly. I've even seen indentations in the abdomen from too-tight pants! Healing is hard work, and many patients report feeling fatigued, even if their bruises have begun to fade.

Now, thanks to computers, faxes, and cell phones, it's much easier for us to work from outside the office. If you're that eager to get back to work, try telecommuting for a couple of days. (Of course, the hazards of some occupations can't be avoided. One of my rhinoplasty patients, a horse trainer, got kicked in the nose only a few weeks after surgery. She wore an ice pack for a day and was fine, but she took a big risk.)

◆ **Housework.** It may be tempting, in the days you're confined to home, to re-arrange your pantry or sweep dust bunnies out from under your bed. But avoid doing anything such as lifting, vacuuming, pushing, or stretching, that might stress your incision and impede your body's ability to heal.

◆ **Smoking.** I can't stress it enough: A cigarette habit greatly compromises healing. Smoking damages skin, keeps incisions from repairing and worsens scarring. Moreover, nicotine, which gets into the bloodstream, can cause blood clots. It's a bad idea to be smoking regularly before you have surgery, and an even worse idea after.

◆ **Exposure to sun.** Going in the sun after surgery is a terrible idea. Sun exposure boosts melanin production, causing hyperpigmentation, and a sunburn anywhere near the affected area causes undue stress. That said, many patients are eager to hit the beach, pool, and tennis court to flaunt their new recontoured bodies. That's understandable, but be smart. I once did eleventh-hour liposuction on a bride-to-be (two weeks before her wedding she could no longer fit into her dress). The hitch was that she had planned a tropical honeymoon. I didn't forbid her from going to the beach, but advised her to stay under an umbrella as much as possible and to use an effective sunscreen, preferably one containing zinc oxide.

◆ **Travel.** Any time the extremities swell, you're at risk for *venus thrombosis*, a clotting of the veins that occurs when you're stationary for long periods of time. Still, patients come to me from all over the world and hop on a plane home a few days after their surgeries. I tell them to be sensible. That may mean splurging on a business- or first-class ticket rather than squeezing into a coach seat. When flying, get up and walk around every hour or so to prevent blood from pooling. And drink plenty of water to keep the body and skin hydrated.

◆ **Sex.** If your surgery was on an area that can be compromised during sex—near the abdomen, breasts, thighs, or groin—the incisions are at risk for being stressed. As with exercise, you must also avoid elevating your blood pressure for a couple of weeks. You needn't abstain from sex for longer than that, though. Once, I neglected to discuss with a breast reduction patient the exact duration of the embargo. When she came in a couple of months later for a follow-up visit, she asked when she could start having sex again. Poor woman—that's not an oversight I've made since!

◆ **Hair styling.** Incisions on and around the face and neck shouldn't be subjected to harsh chemicals from dyes and sprays for four to six weeks. Avoid using a hair dryer for the same time period. The skin around the hairline can be numb after surgery, and you risk burning yourself.

◆ **Shaving.** Men who have had facial surgery (and women who've had an implant inserted through their armpits) should take care not to shave too soon after surgery, because the area around the scar may remain numb for several weeks and they can nick themselves without feeling it.

PATIENT, HEAL THYSELF

No matter how well a surgeon does his or her part, you must be cautious and nurture yourself throughout your healing. I don't expect you to follow my directions to a T, but you can use my recommendations to make the lifestyle changes needed to keep your recovery a top priority.

The next step in embracing a life of cosmetic wellness is to consider the whole-body picture and not just treat the symptoms. If you take a holistic approach to your healing, your body will bounce back better and quicker. In the following section, you'll find suggestions for being pro-active in getting yourself back into peak shape.

The Exercise Connection

As I've said, exercise promotes healing. In the days following surgery, light exercise helps control swelling and allows the tissues to heal without inhibiting mobility. (Keep in mind, though, that you don't want to break a sweat until after your incision heals, because this promotes infection.) In the next few weeks and months, exercise can help restore your strength and promote a more positive outlook. This is not the time to start an aggressive exercise regimen if you've never had one. But if you're accustomed to working out, you'll feel a lot better if you can start moving again soon. I have a small gym in my office, and I often recommend that patients come to see my exercise trainer, who can tailor a program to their needs.

A Few Activities I Recommend

◆ **Walking.** Brisk walking boosts circulation and improves healing. With most procedures, you can begin as early as the day after surgery.

◆ **Swimming.** Swimming can be especially good for breast implant patients, because the arm movements help to prevent capsulation. Be sure your incisions have totally healed before immersing yourself in water.

◆ **Bicycling.** As long as your surgery wasn't a buttock lift, biking is a great way to get aerobic exercise with minimal jiggling and stress on your incisions.

◆ **Weight training.** I encourage all liposuction patients to take up a weight-training program. Surgery is only part of the answer to creating the body of your dreams. The only way to get definition in those areas that have been lipoed, from abdomen to arms, is to strength train. And no, lifting weights does not make women "bulky." An added bonus: Muscle tissue burns twice as many calories as fat does when your body is resting. A note for breast implant patients: My experience shows that it's beneficial to lift one- to two-pound weights within a few days of surgery to diminish the chance of capsular contracture. Ask your doctor about this before proceeding.

A Few Activities to Avoid for a While

◆ **Yoga.** Yes, it's low-impact and a great way to relax. But face-surgery patients should swear off yoga for a few weeks, as many positions require inversion, which is terrible for your incisions.

◆ **Jogging.** Vigorous jostling is disruptive to healing. Lipo and lift patients should wait at least four weeks, until skin re-adheres, to resume jogging.

◆ **Step aerobics.** Breast-surgery patients should avoid step classes in particular for the same reasons they should avoid jogging.

◆ **Tennis, basketball, and other ball/"contact" sports.** Face-surgery patients shouldn't risk getting beaned. Also, the vigorous darting, jumping, and sprinting involved in these sports are stressful to any type of incision.

Food, Glorious Food

Nutrition plays a large role in the healing process. For several weeks following surgery, stick to a bland diet so that you don't trigger inflammation or cause indigestion (particularly if you've had anything done to your midsection, such as liposuction or a tummy tuck). Also, this is no time to try to lose weight. As it heals, your body will crave nutrition. It will need ample protein, which contains the amino acids used in building and repairing tissue. The best sources of protein are meat, fish, poultry, dairy products, soy products, or legumes. Because protein-rich foods also tend to be fatty, some patients may avoid them, especially while they are less physically active. But even if you choose to skip meat, which can be hard to digest, don't skimp on other sources of protein.

There are many vitamins and minerals that promote healing. They include:

- **Vitamin C.** Early sailors who spent months on the high seas would get connective-tissue diseases because they were deprived of vitamin C, which aids collagen formation. Vitamin C is easily digested in supplement form, but you can also find it in citrus, broccoli, peppers, and brussels sprouts.

- **Vitamin A.** Your body uses vitamin A, and its precursor beta carotene, for growth, healthy skin, and cells that line the body's openings (mouth, nose, lungs, etc.). Good food sources include liver, eggs, butter, and orange or yellow vegetables.

- **Vitamin B.** A deficiency in B vitamins (riboflavin, thiamin, and niacin) can inhibit blood formation and collagen production. Vitamin B–rich foods include green leafy vegetables, whole-grain breads and cereals, legumes, nuts, and eggs.

- **Vitamin K.** A vitamin we don't hear a lot about, K helps the blood to clot. It is found in cabbage, cauliflower, spinach, and other leafy greens.

- **Iron.** Low iron levels are not uncommon after surgery. Your body needs iron to help the blood transport oxygen. Replenish your stores with animal products, such as red meat, fish or poultry, and leafy greens (such as kale and mustard greens) and legumes (beans and peas). Iron-fortified cereals are also a good source.

- **Zinc.** Depressed zinc levels may affect wound-healing by inhibiting the creation of fibroblasts, the cells that lay down collagen. High-protein foods such as beef, pork, and lamb contain high amounts of zinc. Other good zinc sources are peanuts and other legumes.

Some Foods to Avoid After Surgery

◆ **Salt.** Because it encourages the body to retain water and makes blood circulation sluggish, salt can increase inflammation. Stay away from salty foods like pretzels, pizza, and some soups (chicken soup may be great for a cold, but it's not recommended post-surgery). Processed foods such as cheeses and canned sauces can contain heaps of hidden salt. I've also found that canned tuna fish can promote inflammation and a tingling in the salivary glands. Check the labels for salt content.

◆ **Spicy foods.** In New York, at least, the first thing people want to do when they're ready to go back to a normal diet is to order out for Chinese food. But spices and some additives, especially monosodium glutamate (MSG), can increase inflammation. Also, sour foods can stimulate the salivary glands, causing swelling in the mouth.

◆ **Alcohol.** Some patients report that the tannins in red wine can trigger inflammation in the mouth. All types of alcohol should be avoided while you're on antibiotics.

Give Yourself a Mental "Lift"

Not everyone is thrilled with their surgery when they get home. More often than not, in fact, patients report that the first time they look in the mirror they feel terror, revulsion, and everything in between. "I did reel back," recalls Julia of her mini-lift and eye job. "Early on, you have to live on belief that what you did is going to be great for you."

Your frame of mind affects your recovery. A positive attitude not only keeps you motivated to take good care of yourself as you heal, but helps you get the physical results you were seeking. Carry yourself with pride and confidence, and that positive energy will draw favorable attention to whatever it is you have changed, be it your face, breasts, arms, or hips. A few ideas for creating, and keeping, an upbeat frame of mind:

◆ If possible, avoid friends or family members who disapproved of your surgery. Their observations, though well intended, will only fill your head with doubt.

◆ Be patient. It can take up to three weeks for most bruising and swelling to dissipate, and the healing continues for weeks after that. It's pointless to cry over your new nose before then; it's not the nose you'll end up with.

◆ Keep a "before" picture nearby for reference. If you're doubting your reason for going through with surgery, just take a gander at those heavy arms, or flat chest, or crow's-feet, and you'll be reminded of what you were so unhappy about.

◆ Have a support system in place. For those who are always in control of every aspect of their lives, feeling out of control is unsettling. It's helpful and calming to have a safety net of caring friends and family who can help you manage the details of your life, from running errands to paying bills.

◆ Treat your pain. Sometimes a patient's doubt is the result of feeling overwhelmed by pain. Everyone experiences pain differently; some report almost none after major surgeries while others are laid low for days. Talk to your doctor about ways to manage pain *before* it becomes a problem.

Although you may not want to hear this when you're the one enduring it, the healing process has become much easier, shorter, and less painful than it was even ten years ago. One thing remains the same, though: During and certainly after the healing, you're left looking better, younger, and healthier than you did before you took the courageous step of making this change to your life. If you take control of your healing with the same spirit of initiative and optimism that led you to pursue surgery, then your recovery will inevitably proceed more smoothly.

You Own Your Body.
It Doesn't Own You.

As a physician who loves what she does and the positive changes her work engenders, I'm admittedly biased when it comes to evaluating cosmetic surgery. As with most anything, there are pros and cons. Obviously, I think that for the vast majority of patients, the pros far outweigh the cons. Choosing a procedure to fix a long-term problem that has negatively affected how you feel about yourself and interact with the world—to my mind, that's the definition of good mental health. There's nothing "cosmetic" about that, or vain, or neurotic. It's practical, constructive, forward-moving, pro-active, and self-affirming. In short, it improves your life and makes you happier about things—or, at the very least (though there's hardly anything "least" about it), it diminishes or outright removes your unhappiness about some specific thing: thunder thighs, wrinkles, jowls, a beer gut, or a flat or too-prominent chest. That capacity to change one's whole outlook is perhaps the most wonderful "pro" of cosmetic surgery that I see and live with every day. That's why I'm an unabashed cheerleader of my discipline, so long as patient and doctor follow a common objective with intelligence, level-headedness, thoroughness, and a positive attitude.

There is, of course, a small percentage of people, some of whom have been written about in the press, who have pursued plastic surgery solutions but shouldn't have. These are the cosmetic surgery "junkie," on the one hand, and the impossible-to-satisfy patient on the other (though the categories overlap). Neither of these types, in my opinion, can achieve a satisfactory plastic surgery result. The cosmetic surgery junkie is constantly going for consultations about this body-part fix or that, then undergoing the procedure, then moving on to another fix, and another, and another. Perhaps he or she enjoys the feeling of connectedness that comes with a visit to the doctor; that's not uncommon. I have no problem with a patient who, having enjoyed a great result on one part of the body, wants to enjoy that same great feeling about another. Many of my patients start with one procedure, having got past the trepidation of undergoing plastic surgery to see how their looks and life changed for the better, then come back to fix something else. But the junkie, who can't feel satisfied if she or he is not in the midst of a new transformation of the body, is not always easy to spot.

Recently, a New Yorker addicted to plastic surgery (she'd undergone more than fifty operations) sued her surgeon because she felt that he should have refused to perform the last of her surgeries (he didn't do all the previous ones) and should instead have referred her to a psychiatrist for her mental problems. It's no accident, in my opinion, that she sued only after undergoing an operation whose result she was not entirely happy with—a tummy tuck—even though the doctor had, according to court documents, discussed with her extensively the risks and resulting scar of the procedure, as well as other options. The lawsuit was tossed out; the court found no definitive link between her depression and her obsession.

The fundamental difference between the cosmetic surgery junkie and the well-adjusted patient who undergoes several procedures, then, is that the former hovers in a state of perpetual dissatisfaction, whereas the latter is simply building one satisfaction on top of another. That's healthy.

Dissatisfaction with oneself is at the root of the other personality type who should not get plastic surgery; I mean those who suffer from a clinical affliction known as Body Dysmorphic Disorder (BDD). Those who experience this rare psychiatric disorder are preoccupied with small and imagined flaws in their appearance; they think about these flaws three to eight hours a day, on average. Among other behavioral markers for those with BDD is, not surprisingly, dissatisfaction with surgical results. The American Society for Aesthetic Plastic Surgery (ASAPS) recently stated that patients suffering from BDD are inappropriate candidates for plastic surgery.

Can I spot these types? Not necessarily. But often I can tell, by questions that prospective patients ask in consultation, when trouble is brewing. One candidate came in and said, "My cheeks are flat and I'd like them to be a little plumper." That's reasonable, and presents a problem I can correct. However, another candidate, pointing to her face, once said to me, "You see this line here? I hate it. Can you pull everything tight enough so it'll be gone? And this line right here? Also, this line . . . ?" To me, that spells trouble. I told her I could improve the appearance of her wrinkles, but that they wouldn't completely disappear. Dissatisfied with my answer, she sought out a different surgeon.

When dealing with patients who have a healthy body image, I affirm all the positives of what they're doing. I also make sure they understand that I, like any surgeon, can only do my very best. I explain, too, that skin, and bodies, and the world in general, are not perfect. I make sure that a lipo candidate with poor skin tone knows she may have more irregularity than she'd hoped for. She must decide whether losing the fat is an acceptable trade-off for the scar, albeit a tiny one. Is it worth it? That's what we try to answer beforehand. *Was* it worth it? That's something the patient has to answer after the fact. If you're armed with realistic expectations and knowledge of what's going to happen, then you're presumably in an excellent position to make the right decision. I don't want to operate on a patient who I know, going in, won't be happy with the results.

Ironically, because advances in my discipline have been so rapid, numerous, and dramatic, patients in the last several years may have become less, not more, realistic about what they can expect from surgery. As more and more people go for nonsurgical lunchtime fixes—a collagen or Botox injection here, a laser spot removal there—with such great and immediate results, they've come to expect that surgery, too, should provide them with exactly what they want, fast, and with minimal hassle. That's not the case. As I've said before, *it's surgery*. Your looks and outlook will improve, often greatly. But you must temper your expectations.

Many patients who obsess before surgery (in Chapter 1, I outlined many of the plaguing questions), obsess *after* surgery, too. *What did I just do?* they wonder. *Why did I do it? Was that the biggest mistake I ever made?* Keep the following in mind to help diminish some of the sting you may feel post-surgery:

◆ **The result you see right after surgery will improve.** Bruising and swelling have yet to go down, and "settling" has yet to occur. Give it time.

◆ **Remember what you looked like before the change.** Keep a "before" picture handy. It's amazing how quickly patients can forget how bad they felt—for years—about the very thing that inspired them to pursue plastic surgery. It's crucial to recall as much of the unhappiness you're *not* feeling anymore as it is the contentment you *are* feeling.

◆ **The disruption in my life is temporary.** During recovery, even a relatively speedy one, it's easy to melt down over the suspension of one's daily routine. In the long run, this "endless" period will be but a blip on the screen. Take advantage of the downtime (from work and day-to-day stress) to do things you rarely get the chance to do: Lie down and listen to a favorite CD, rent an old movie, or take a leisurely walk through a museum if you feel presentable (or along a lamplit sidewalk, if you don't).

◆ **Given my courage to change my looks, who knows what I'm capable of accomplishing now?** You made a bold decision to have surgery. Perhaps that's what you needed to break through and give yourself the strength to pursue more ambitious goals.

The great benefit of cosmetic surgery comes not merely from, say, fixing your breasts or erasing worry lines from your face, troublesome as those problems may have been. The true benefit comes from the more profound changes my patients make to their lives *after* surgery, because having the surgery helped them see that improvement—genuine, palpable, near-term improvement—is possible. They now want to do everything they can to help that along.

That, in a nutshell, is "cosmetic wellness." When my patients come out of their surgical experience thrilled—and they usually do—they are more likely, perhaps for the first time in their lives, to follow a skin-care regimen, to eat healthier foods, to exercise regularly, to sleep longer and better, and to quit bad habits (such as smoking, nail biting, or drinking too much). Having just made their situation so much better; they have every incentive to build on improving their lives. The notion that they can now take control of their looks and lives merely by altering everyday habits empowers them.

I've seen this transformation happen countless times among my patients. One after the other will tell you that the benefits they enjoy now reach much deeper and further than tighter buns or flatter bellies or bigger-cup-sized breasts. The change in their looks improves the essence of their lives.

I recently got a note from a patient on whom I'd performed a face-lift. She wrote, "Should someone ask what you do for a living, you might answer, 'I create possibility.' "

But plastic surgeons don't create possibility—you do. We're just here to help you to become whoever it is you want to be.

GLOSSARY

AHA (Alpha-hydroxy acid). A superficial peel, or exfoliant, derived from natural sources such as fruit and milk that helps shed superficial skin cells, leaving a smoother complexion.

Anesthesia. Loss of bodily sensation caused by the administration of a drug. Types of anesthetic generally used in plastic surgery procedures include local, local with sedation, and general.

Autologous fat transfer. A procedure in which one's own fat is liposuctioned out of the buttocks, abdomen, or thigh areas and injected in the face for plumping up and eliminating wrinkles.

Body Dysmorphic Disorder (BDD). A psychiatric disorder in which sufferers are preoccupied with small or imagined flaws in their appearance, and have exceedingly unrealistic hopes for the outcome of their surgery.

Botox (Botulinum Toxin Type A). A bacteria-derived, naturally occurring chemical that, when injected into the forehead and neck muscles, temporarily paralyzes them and erases wrinkles caused by their use. It often takes a few days to see the effect of Botox.

Breast lift (mastopexy). A surgical procedure that removes excess skin and tissue of the breast and repositions the nipple in a higher location. This is often done after nursing or gravity has pulled the breasts down.

Breast reduction (mammoplasty). A surgical procedure performed to reduce the size of the breasts by removing excess skin and fat.

Cannula. A small probing tube used to remove fat by liposuction.

Capsular contracture. The formation of scar tissue around a breast implant; the breast feels painful, tight, and hard.

Chemical peel. A face peel, using phenol, trichloroacetic acid, or glycolic acid, that removes unwanted skin layers to promote the regrowth of new, smoother skin.

CO_2 laser. An ablative laser that works to remove wrinkles by vaporizing the top layer of skin using carbon dioxide. May leave the skin looking red and flaky.

Collagen. A strong, fibrous protein derived from cow skin that is injected into wrinkles and lines to temporarily plump them up. *See* Human Collagen.

Dermabrasion. A surgery to smooth out facial scars by removing the skin's outer layers using an abrasive tool. May leave the face red and raw. *See* Microdermabrasion.

Edema. Excessive accumulation of fluid in the tissues, causing swelling.

Endermologie. A nonsurgical technique that uses electrical heating pulses to massage cellulite; patients must undergo numerous treatments before results become apparent. Although best used in conjunction with liposuction, the technique's effectiveness is an issue of debate.

Endoscope. A tube-shaped probe with a microscopic optical instrument that is inserted through a small incision during surgery, permitting the surgeon to see and perform cosmetic procedures such as forehead lifts and breast implants. This typically reduces post-operative swelling, bruising, and discomfort.

Endoscopic forehead lift. A surgical brow lift that is done by inserting an endoscope through three tiny incisions at the hairline.

Erbium laser. An ablative laser that removes wrinkles when its energy is absorbed by the water in skin cells, causing shrinkage and collagen regeneration.

Eyelid lift (blepharoplasty). Cosmetic surgery to tighten sagging and wrinkled eyelids by removing fat and/or skin, usually to reduce signs of aging.

Face-lift (rhytidectomy). An operation that repositions the skin to remove creases and tighten the lower half of the face, thus countering the effects of aging.

Facial implant surgery. A surgical operation to insert bone, cartilage, or synthetic material into the face to balance features such as the lips, chin, cheeks, or nose.

Fascia. Fibrous tissue found beneath the skin that encloses muscles and separates the tissue layers of the body.

Forehead lift (coronal lift). A traditional facial rejuvenation surgery that diminishes wrinkles, frown lines between the brows, and other signs of aging on the forehead. *See* Endoscopic forehead lift.

Glycolic acid. A fruit acid used in chemical peels; also an ingredient in skin-care products employed to rejuvenate facial skin.

Gynecomastia. A condition in which there is excessive breast development in males, without hormonal imbalance.

Hair removal lasers. Lasers (types include Diode, Long Pulse, Ruby) that perform photoepilation by directing light at the melanin in hair.

Hematoma. Blood collection under the skin, a common post-operative occurrence that often resolves on its own but can be surgically removed.

Hemorrhage. Heavy, uncontrolled bleeding.

Human Collagen. An injectable filler derived from cadavers that is used to plump the face and minimize wrinkles and lines.

Hyaluronic acid. An injectable filler derived from connective fibers in plants and from bacteria. Easy to inject and longer lasting then collagen, it has been used for years in Europe but has yet to be approved for use in the U.S. by the FDA.

Hydroquinone. A class of chemicals used to bleach skin.

Hyperpigmentation. Excessive discoloration of the skin, often caused by overexposure to the sun.

Implant. A surgically placed insert, often made of synthetic material, that is used to correct bodily deficiencies or aesthetic imbalance.

Intense Pulsed Light (IPL). A wrinkle-reducing treatment that uses multiple wavelengths of light to trigger collagen growth and treat pigmentation issues such as rosacea and age spots. Because it is gentle and non-specifically directed, it may require multiple sessions to produce results.

Keloid. Red, fibrous scar tissue that forms at the site of an incision due to an overproduction of collagen.

Laser. An acronym for Light Amplification by Stimulated Emission of Radiation, this concentrated beam is used in a variety of ways, including to make incisions that barely bleed, to resurface skin, and to remove surface veins and wrinkles.

Laser resurfacing (laser peel). A facial rejuvenation surgery that uses a laser beam to eliminate or modify skin defects. Laser resurfacing treatments can be ablative (taking off the top layer of skin, which can result in redness and scarring) or non-ablative light touch. Laser types include Nd: YAG, Alexandrite, and Pulsed Dye.

Light touch laser (Nd: YAG, Alexandrite, Pulsed Dye). A non-ablative laser that only imperceptibly removes the top layer of skin, smoothing wrinkles and stimulating collagen growth. Ideal for mild to moderate wrinkling.

Liposuction. A cosmetic procedure that removes excess fat by suctioning it out of the body using a cannula and vacuum.

Local anesthetic. An agent that, when injected into the body, causes a loss of sensation without loss of consciousness. It is often given in conjunction with a mild relaxant.

Melanin. A naturally occurring pigment that protects the skin from ultraviolet (UV) rays.

Microdermabrasion. A skin-smoothing technique in which fine crystals are sprayed at the skin, removing the top, dead layer. It is most effective on fine lines, large pores, and adult acne.

Mini-lift (mini-rhytidectomy). A facial procedure for patients with minimal signs of aging, in which the skin and tissues are lifted and redraped from the mid-face to the chin or neck.

Nasolabial fold. The creases extending from the side of the nostril to the corner of the mouth.

Otoplasty. A procedure to tack protruding ears permanently into normal position.

PAL (power-assisted liposuction). A liposuction technique in which the cannula powers through tissue, and vacuums out fat and fibrous tissue with minimal effort and little risk of burning.

Phenol. A strong chemical used in resurfacing the skin.

Retin-A. A medication derived from vitamin A, prescribed to treat acne and reduce wrinkles.

Rhinoplasty (nose job). Surgery of the bone and cartilage to reshape the contour or change the size of the nose.

SAL (suction-assisted liposuction). A traditional liposuction method in which undesired fat is removed through a cannula attached to a vacuum, inserted in a tiny incision.

Skin resurfacing. Any surgical procedure that removes top skin layers to produce new skin, thus diminishing acne scars, wrinkles, and sun damage. *See also* Laser resurfacing, Dermabrasion, Microdermabrasion.

Spider veins (telangiectasias). Nonessential dilated veins visible through the surface of the skin. They can be eliminated using laser treatment.

Spot removal lasers. Lasers that remove blemishes and dark spots by vaporizing the pigment in skin.

Suture. To close a wound surgically by sewing or stapling it.

Tumescent liposuction. A fat-suctioning technique in which a dilute anesthetic solution is injected into the skin, causing the treated area to balloon in order to simplify the removal of fat and ensure minimal patient discomfort.

Tummy tuck (abdominoplasty). An operation to flatten the stomach by removing excess skin and fat.

Twilight sedation ("twilight sleep"). A combination of medications (Versed and Propythal) transferred through an intravenous tube that leaves the patient in a tranquil, relaxed state of mind without rendering him or her unconscious. The patient is always breathing on his/her own, without a tube, and is usually left without any groggy after-effects.

UAL (ultrasound-assisted liposuction). A liposuction technique that uses sound waves to break down fat while removing it. This technique ensures minimal blood and tissue loss, because it removes fat discriminately.

INDEX

Fellows of the American College of Surgeons (FACS), 49
Food and Drug Administration (FDA), 23, 58, 81, 84–86, 89, 147, 149
forehead:
  facial surgery and, 103, 105–6, 109, 116–18, 120–25, 128–29
  quick fixes for wrinkles on, 86–87, 89
forehead lifts (coronal lifts), 5–7, 25, 29, 31–32
  choosing doctors and, 54, 56
  cost of, 20
  endoscopic, xiv–xv, 14, 17, 31–32, 37, 105, 109, 116–17, 120–25, 128–29, 216, 219–20
  eyelid surgery with, 128–29
  incisions in, 122–23, 219–20
  for men, 216, 219–20
  for migraine relief, 122
  mini-, 7
  mini-face-lifts with, 219
  problems treated by, 109
  recovery after, 123
  right time for, 37
  side effects of, 123–24
frown lines, 108–9
  quick fixes for, 75, 79, 84, 86
full body lifts, 207–8

gigantomastia, 169–70
glycolic acids, 8, 27, 67, 69, 193, 227, 234
Goretex, 85, 88, 137
gynecomastia:
  cost of treatment for, 20
  liposuction for, 189, 224–25
  surgery for, 223–26

hair, hairline, 18
  facial surgery and, 110, 113–15, 119, 121–25
  healing and, 231, 236–37, 243
  laser removal of, 20, 40, 76, 91, 96–97, 219, 226
  length of, 115
  loss of, 113, 124
  and procedures for men, 214–15, 217, 219–20, 222, 225–26
  transplantation of, 20
hands, 10, 91–92
healing, 8, 12, 15, 17–18, 22–23, 31–32, 35, 229–48
  and advances in cosmetic surgery, xiv–xv
  after body recontouring, 176, 179–80, 182, 184, 188–93, 195, 201–2, 204–5, 207–10
  breast surgery and, 146, 152–55, 157, 164, 171, 173, 231, 233, 235, 237, 239, 242–45, 247–48
  bruising and, 229, 236–37, 242, 248, 252

choosing doctors and, 48–49, 52–53, 55
facial surgery and, 104–8, 111–14, 118–20, 123, 125–26, 128, 130, 132–34, 138–40, 231–32, 234, 237–39, 241–43, 245, 247
at home, 237–40
infections and, 232–33, 235–37, 240, 244
and non-ablative lasers, 77
nurturing yourself throughout, 243–48
partners in, 232–33
and procedures for men, 216, 219–22, 225
scars in, 233–36, 240, 243
skin care and, 66
before surgery, 229–32
taking charge of, 237–43
and timing of surgery, 42–43
hips, 3–4, 88
  beauty standards and, 26
  healing and, 247
  liposuction for, 37–38, 183–88, 196, 224
  and procedures for men, 219, 224
  and quick fixes for wrinkles, 81–82
  recontouring of, 175–78, 183–88, 196, 198
housework, 242
Hyaluronic acid, 85, 89
hyperpigmentation, 93, 242
  body recontouring and, 193–94
hypersensitivity, 192

infection, infections, 23
  body recontouring and, 193, 195, 207, 211
  breast surgery and, 151, 158, 164
  facial surgery and, 112, 115, 119–20, 123–24, 126, 130, 139, 142
  healing and, 232–33, 235–37, 240, 244
  and procedures for men, 216
  of scars, 235
inferior pedicle breast lifts, 163–64
inferior pedicle breast reductions, 170
inframammary incisions, 153
Intense Pulsed Light (IPL), 77, 95
Internet, 51, 57–58
iron, 246

jogging, 245
jowls, 9, 107–8, 249
  body recontouring and, 188
  facial surgery and, 104–5, 107, 117, 125, 131, 177
  and patient age, 40
  and procedures for men, 217, 219–20, 226
  quick fixes for, 78–79

keloidal scars, 115, 165–66, 193, 211, 233–35
knees, 177–79, 189, 191

cost of, 76, 97
facial surgery and, 115
for men, 226
right time for, 39–40
for scars, 235
for wrinkles, 74–76, 78–79
migraines, 122
moisturizers, moisturizing, 27, 63, 65, 69, 71,
227, 234–35
mouth:
facial surgery and, 109, 114, 132–33, 140
healing and, 247
quick fixes for wrinkles around, 74–75, 79,
81, 84, 86, 88
muscle enhancement, 226–27
Myobloc, 87

nasolabial fold, 30, 108–9
facial surgery and, 109, 117, 133
quick fixes for, 75, 82–84, 86, 88–89
National Institutes of Health, 148
neck, 173, 193
breast surgery and, 150, 167
facial surgery and, 103, 106–7, 109, 111–13
healing and, 231, 234, 237–39, 241
liposuction for, 14–15, 18, 104, 188, 213, 217,
220
and procedures for men, 213, 217, 219–22
quick fixes for blemishes on, 93
quick fixes for wrinkles on, 76, 79, 86, 89
neck lifts, xv, 5, 22–23, 188
chin augmentations with, 131
face-lifts and, 111–13, 116, 125–26
and getting results you want, 30, 33
healing after, 125–26, 238
for men, 221–22
patient age for, 37
problems treated by, 109
procedure for, 125
side effects of, 113
neck lipectomies, 15, 107, 188
chin augmentations with, 131
for men, 213, 220–21
problems treated by, 109
procedure for, 125
recovery after, 125–26
nerve damage, 23, 124
nose, noses, 3, 12, 13, 25, 28
carbon-copy, 137
changing angle of, 140
facial surgery and, 109, 121, 131, 135–43
malformed shape of, 142
and patient age, 40–41
and procedures for men, 220
quick fixes for blemishes on, 93

quick fixes for wrinkles around, 75, 82–84,
86, 88–89
smoothing bumps and softening tips of, 139
nose jobs (rhinoplasties), 7, 12, 25, 28, 33,
135–43
choosing doctors and, 47, 56
closed, 136, 138
cost of, 19, 21, 32, 137–38
healing after, 17, 119, 138–40, 237–38,
241–42
incisions in, 138
open, 135–36, 138
right time for, 37, 43
side effects of, 141–42
numbness, 218
body recontouring and, 193–94, 209–10
breast surgery and, 157–58, 165, 169
facial surgery and, 113, 122–24, 126, 132,
140–41
healing and, 243
and procedures for men, 220, 225
nutrition, 27, 110, 252–53
body recontouring and, 176, 178–79, 190,
195, 197, 200
breast surgery and, 146, 152
cosmetic wellness and, xviii–xix
healing and, 230–33, 238–39, 245–47
and patient age, 39–41
and procedures for men, 219
skin care and, 65

overweight:
body recontouring and, 175, 178–80, 183,
185, 189, 196–200, 208
breast surgery and, 167–68
and procedures for men, 213, 225

pain, 10, 14–15, 17, 33, 96
and advances in cosmetic surgery, xiv–xv
body recontouring and, 180, 188, 192–93,
204, 209–10
breast surgery and, 146, 150, 152–54, 156–59,
164, 167–68, 171, 173
choosing doctors and, 45, 55
facial surgery and, 103, 112–13, 119–20,
122–23, 125–26, 134, 139, 141
healing and, 229, 232–33, 238–39, 241, 248
and procedures for men, 216, 227
and quick fixes for wrinkles, 74
paralysis, 114
pectoral implants, 227
periareolar (pursestring) incisions, 153, 157–58,
162, 164, 170
phenol, 67
photo-epilation, 96

ABOUT THE AUTHORS

MICHELLE COPELAND, D.M.D., M.D., received both doctorates from Harvard University and currently holds the position of Assistant Professor of Surgery at the Mount Sinai School of Medicine, New York University. As a member of the Medical Health Advisory Board for the Society for the Advancement of Women's Health Research, Dr. Copeland advises Congress on health issues affecting women. She has authored numerous scientific articles and appeared frequently in magazines and on television, including *The New York Times, Allure*, NBC's *Today Show*, and ABC's *Good Morning America*. She practices plastic and reconstructive surgery in Manhattan, where she resides with her husband and two children.

ALEXANDRA S. POSTMAN is a senior features editor at *ELLE* whose work has appeared in several women's magazines, including *Glamour, Mademoiselle*, and *Women's Sports & Fitness*. She lives in Brooklyn with her husband and two sons.